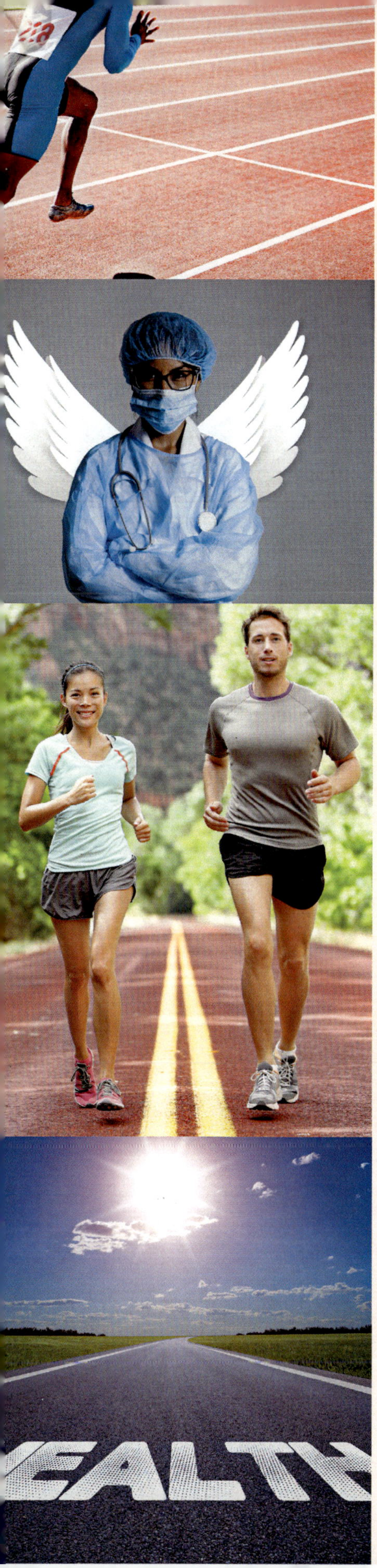

A *Complete* *YEAR* of Health and Wellness Tracker

Vandene Samuel

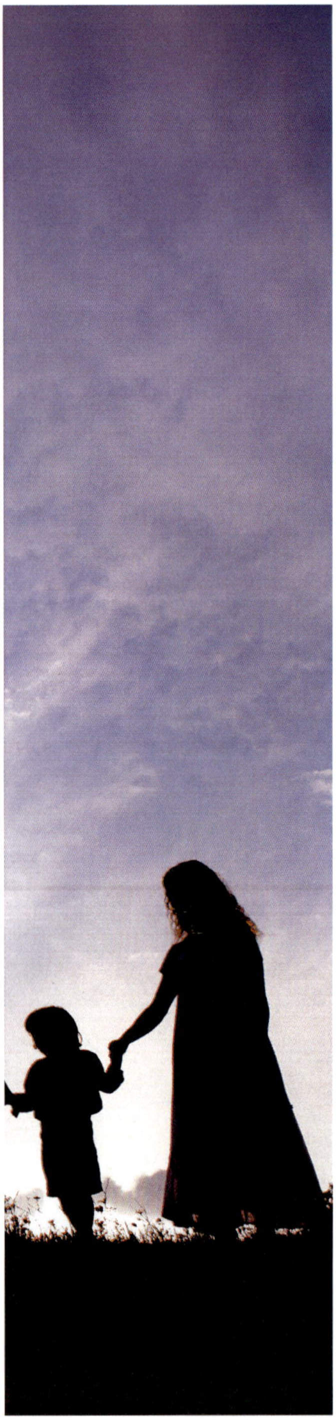

I wrote this book because I wanted to give people a blueprint of how to live an entire year in good health. I am not a doctor, nor am I a nutritionist. I am a mother, a grandmother, a sister, and a wife.

As women, we are the nutritionist for our homes, and if we remain healthy, the whole house will be healthy.

I hope as you go on this journey, you will find out how much you are caring for yourself. It's very important to love one's self, and then that love flows out from you.

Please, share this with your church group, or with your family. Meet up and discuss your progress and revelations. Join my FB Group to keep me updated on your progress.

~ Van

Table of Contents

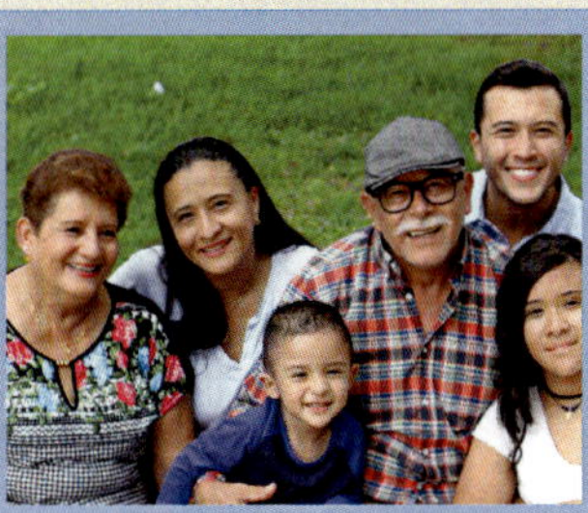
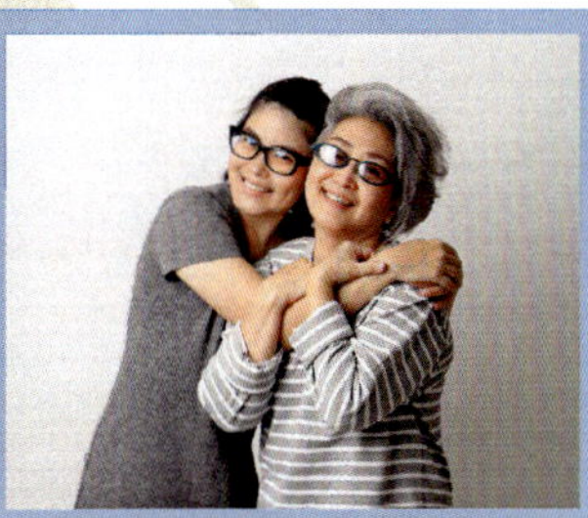

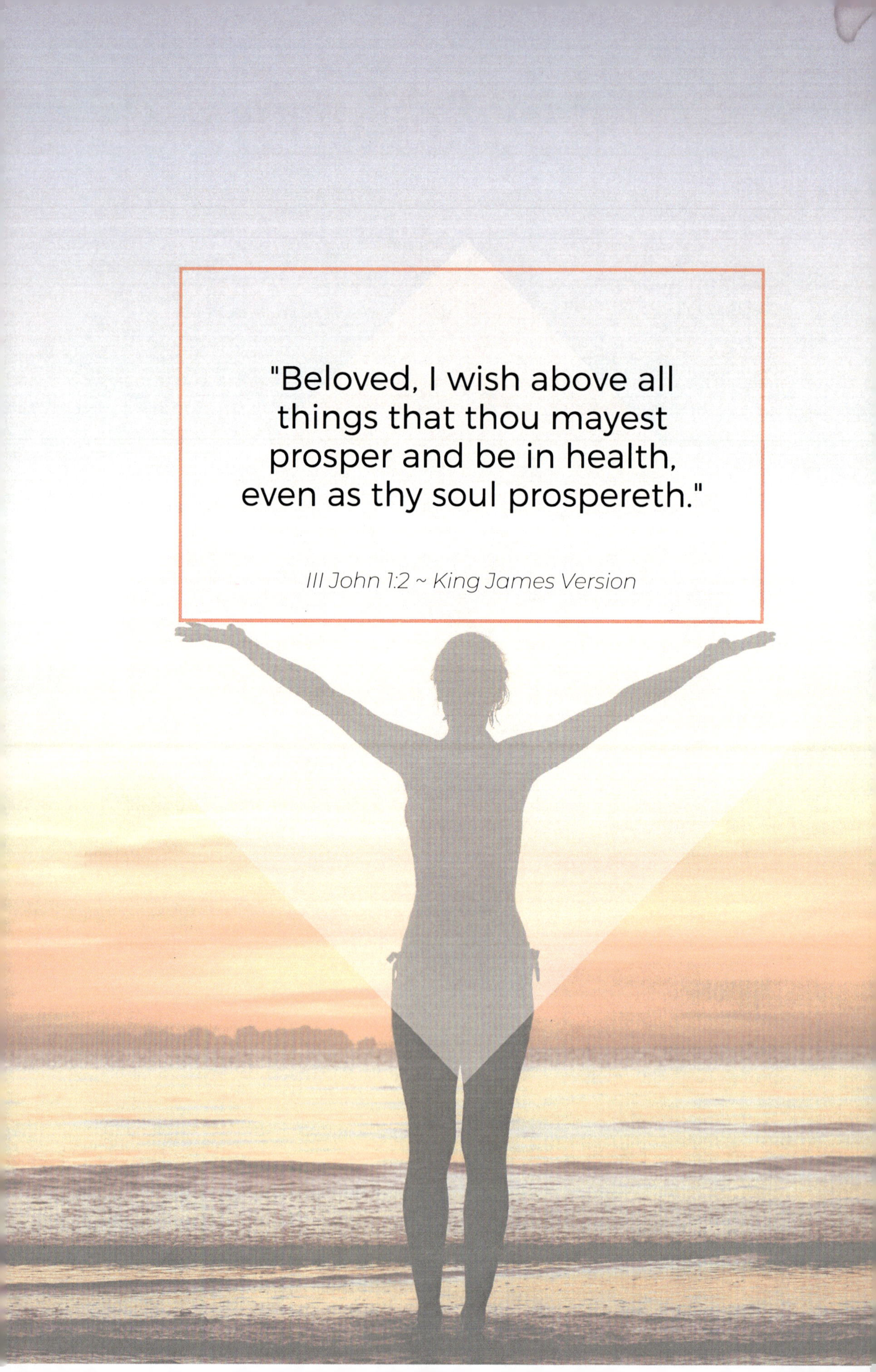

"Beloved, I wish above all things that thou mayest prosper and be in health, even as thy soul prospereth."

III John 1:2 ~ King James Version

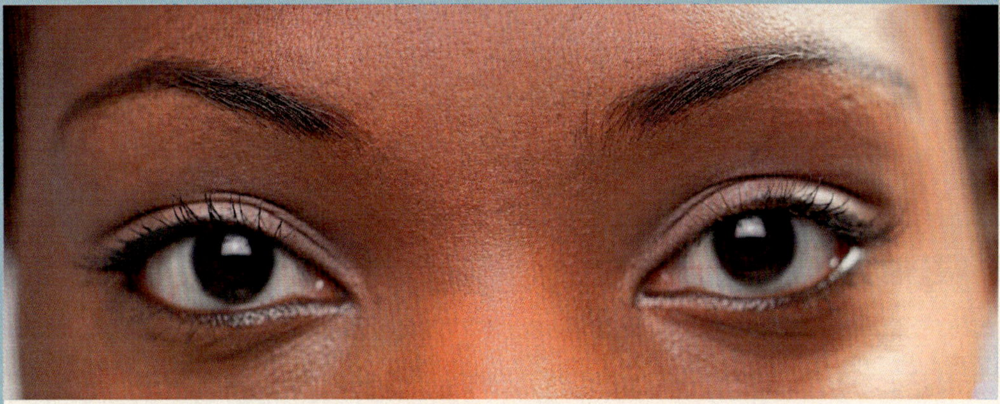

1. EYES

Vision, Cataracts, Glaucoma, Macular Degeneration

They say eyes are the "windows to the soul". It's the way you see the world. As you age, your vision gets worse, even though you are wiser. It's important to think about your eye health before it degenerates.

Eyes are not just about sight, it's also about vision. Your ability to have perspective, imagination, and introspection. Think on the spiritual aspects as well as the physical ones.

Set some goals for the month, and at the end, we will reflect on your progress. You can track your meals, exercise, appointments, and weight goals. Set some spiritual goals too.

GOALS

1. ____
2. ____
3. ____
4. ____
5. ____

> *"The eye is the lamp of the body. So, if your eye is healthy, your whole body will be full of light."*
> *Matthew 6:22*

Monthly Affirmation:

"I am open to seeing things clearly."

Exercise: *Reduce your screen time by 50%. Check your phone and computer for a blue filter setting.*

FOODS to Improve Eye Health:

- **Beans:** Lentils, Black-eyed peas, Kidney Beans, Chickpeas
- **Fat:** Egg
- **Fruit:** Kiwi, Guava, Grapefruit, and Orange
- **Herb:** Green Tea
- **Protein:** Tuna or Trout
- **Nuts:** Sunflower seeds, Almonds
- **Root:** Sweet Potato, Carrot
- **Vegetables:** Kale, Spinach, Collard Greens
- Vitamins: A, E, C, B6, B9, B12, Lutein

JUICE to Improve Eye Health:

Carrot
Ginger
Green Tea

Contact Vandene:
for Local South Florida Delivery
ordersmavis@gmail.com

M.A.V.I.S
Health Drinks

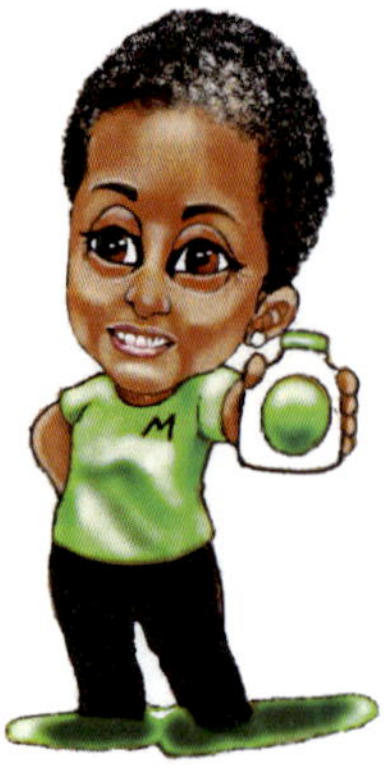

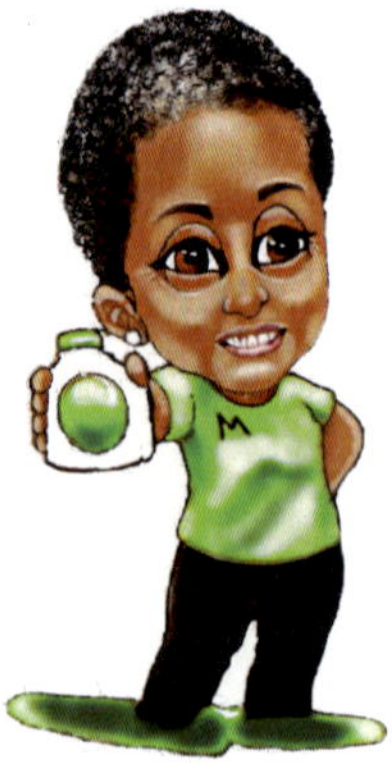

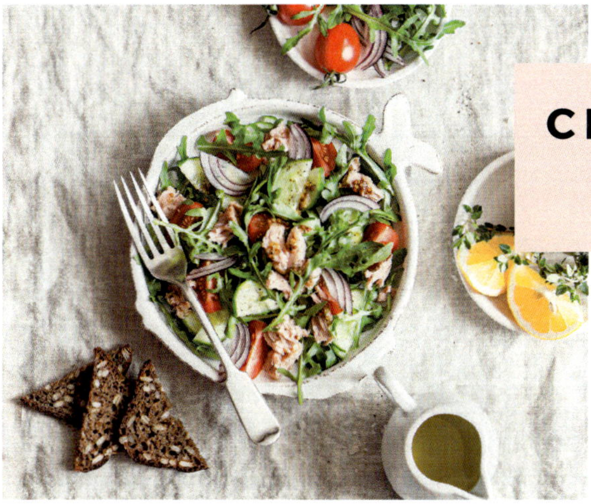

CHICKPEA TUNA KALE SALAD

YIELDS 2 - 3 SERVINGS

PREP TIME: 10 MINS

1 - 6 oz. can of Albacore Tuna in Oil
1 - can of Chickpeas
1 - bunch of Kale
1 - clove of Garlic
2 - tbsps of sliced red onion
1 - lemon
Mayonnaise or salad dressing
2 - tbsps of Olive Oil
1 - dash of ground ginger
1 - dash of ground pepper
1 - dash of mustard

DIRECTIONS:

- Mix Albacore Tuna in oil in a large bowl
- Add Chickpeas (drained0
- Add Sliced Red Onion
- Add Garlic
- Add Lemon Zest
- Add 2 tbsps of lemon juice
- Add Olive Oil
- Add ginger, pepper, and mustard
- Toss thoroughly
- Put over a bed of chopped kale
- Add your favorite mayo or salad dressing
- Chill for 30 minutes (optional)

Medical Appointments

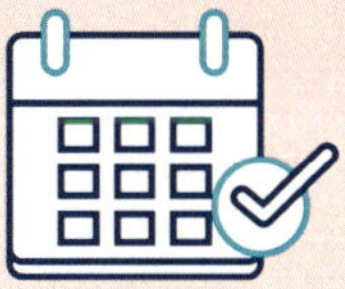

Date/Time	Office

MEAL PLANNER * MONTH ________ YR ______

DAY 1: **MON TUES WED THU FRI SAT SUN** Cal Fat Pro Carbs

B ____________________

L ____________________

S ____________________

D ____________________

DAY 2: **MON TUES WED THU FRI SAT SUN** Cal Fat Pro Carbs

B ____________________

L ____________________

S ____________________

D ____________________

DAY 3: **MON TUES WED THU FRI SAT SUN** Cal Fat Pro Carbs

B ____________________

L ____________________

S ____________________

D ____________________

DAY 4: **MON TUES WED THU FRI SAT SUN** Cal Fat Pro Carbs

B ____________________

L ____________________

S ____________________

D ____________________

DAY 5: **MON TUES WED THU FRI SAT SUN** Cal Fat Pro Carbs

B ____________________

L ____________________

S ____________________

D ____________________

DAY 6: **MON TUES WED THU FRI SAT SUN** Cal Fat Pro Carbs

B ____________________

L ____________________

S ____________________

D ____________________

DAY 7: **MON TUES WED THU FRI SAT SUN** Cal Fat Pro Carbs

B ____________________

L ____________________

S ____________________

D ____________________

ACTIVITY PLANNER * MONTH ______ YR ____

DAY 1: **MON TUES WED THU FRI SAT SUN** *Time* *Calories Burned*

Exercise ____________________

Water ____________ Steps ____________

Sleep ____________ Weight ____________

Stress Level 0 1 2 3 4 5 6 7 8 9 10 11

DAY 2: **MON TUES WED THU FRI SAT SUN** *Time* *Calories Burned*

Exercise ____________________

Water ____________ Steps ____________

Sleep ____________ Weight ____________

Stress Level 0 1 2 3 4 5 6 7 8 9 10 11

DAY 3: **MON TUES WED THU FRI SAT SUN** *Time* *Calories Burned*

Exercise ____________________

Water ____________ Steps ____________

Sleep ____________ Weight ____________

Stress Level 0 1 2 3 4 5 6 7 8 9 10 11

DAY 4: **MON TUES WED THU FRI SAT SUN** *Time* *Calories Burned*

Exercise ____________________

Water ____________ Steps ____________

Sleep ____________ Weight ____________

Stress Level 0 1 2 3 4 5 6 7 8 9 10 11

DAY 5: **MON TUES WED THU FRI SAT SUN** *Time* *Calories Burned*

Exercise ____________________

Water ____________ Steps ____________

Sleep ____________ Weight ____________

Stress Level 0 1 2 3 4 5 6 7 8 9 10 11

DAY 6: **MON TUES WED THU FRI SAT SUN** *Time* *Calories Burned*

Exercise ____________________

Water ____________ Steps ____________

Sleep ____________ Weight ____________

Stress Level 0 1 2 3 4 5 6 7 8 9 10 11

DAY 7: **MON TUES WED THU FRI SAT SUN** *Time* *Calories Burned*

Exercise ____________________

Water ____________ Steps ____________

Sleep ____________ Weight ____________

Stress Level 0 1 2 3 4 5 6 7 8 9 10 11

MEAL PLANNER * MONTH ________ YR ________

DAY 8: **MON TUES WED THU FRI SAT SUN** Cal Fat Pro Carbs

B ____________________

L ____________________

S ____________________

D ____________________

DAY 9: **MON TUES WED THU FRI SAT SUN** Cal Fat Pro Carbs

B ____________________

L ____________________

S ____________________

D ____________________

DAY 10: **MON TUES WED THU FRI SAT SUN** Cal Fat Pro Carbs

B ____________________

L ____________________

S ____________________

D ____________________

DAY 11: **MON TUES WED THU FRI SAT SUN** Cal Fat Pro Carbs

B ____________________

L ____________________

S ____________________

D ____________________

DAY 12: **MON TUES WED THU FRI SAT SUN** Cal Fat Pro Carbs

B ____________________

L ____________________

S ____________________

D ____________________

DAY 13: **MON TUES WED THU FRI SAT SUN** Cal Fat Pro Carbs

B ____________________

L ____________________

S ____________________

D ____________________

DAY 14: **MON TUES WED THU FRI SAT SUN** Cal Fat Pro Carbs

B ____________________

L ____________________

S ____________________

D ____________________

DAY 8: **MON TUES WED THU FRI SAT SUN** *Time* *Calories Burned*

Exercise ______

Water ______ Steps ______

Sleep ______ Weight ______

Stress Level 0 1 2 3 4 5 6 7 8 9 10 11

DAY 9: **MON TUES WED THU FRI SAT SUN** *Time* *Calories Burned*

Exercise ______

Water ______ Steps ______

Sleep ______ Weight ______

Stress Level 0 1 2 3 4 5 6 7 8 9 10 11

DAY 10: **MON TUES WED THU FRI SAT SUN** *Time* *Calories Burned*

Exercise ______

Water ______ Steps ______

Sleep ______ Weight ______

Stress Level 0 1 2 3 4 5 6 7 8 9 10 11

DAY 11: **MON TUES WED THU FRI SAT SUN** *Time* *Calories Burned*

Exercise ______

Water ______ Steps ______

Sleep ______ Weight ______

Stress Level 0 1 2 3 4 5 6 7 8 9 10 11

DAY 12: **MON TUES WED THU FRI SAT SUN** *Time* *Calories Burned*

Exercise ______

Water ______ Steps ______

Sleep ______ Weight ______

Stress Level 0 1 2 3 4 5 6 7 8 9 10 11

DAY 13: **MON TUES WED THU FRI SAT SUN** *Time* *Calories Burned*

Exercise ______

Water ______ Steps ______

Sleep ______ Weight ______

Stress Level 0 1 2 3 4 5 6 7 8 9 10 11

DAY 14: **MON TUES WED THU FRI SAT SUN** *Time* *Calories Burned*

Exercise ______

Water ______ Steps ______

Sleep ______ Weight ______

Stress Level 0 1 2 3 4 5 6 7 8 9 10 11

MEAL PLANNER * MONTH ________ YR ____

DAY 15: MON TUES WED THU FRI SAT SUN Cal Fat Pro Carbs

B ______
L ______
S ______
D ______

DAY 16: MON TUES WED THU FRI SAT SUN Cal Fat Pro Carbs

B ______
L ______
S ______
D ______

DAY 17: MON TUES WED THU FRI SAT SUN Cal Fat Pro Carbs

B ______
L ______
S ______
D ______

DAY 18: MON TUES WED THU FRI SAT SUN Cal Fat Pro Carbs

B ______
L ______
S ______
D ______

DAY 19: MON TUES WED THU FRI SAT SUN Cal Fat Pro Carbs

B ______
L ______
S ______
D ______

DAY 20: MON TUES WED THU FRI SAT SUN Cal Fat Pro Carbs

B ______
L ______
S ______
D ______

DAY 21: MON TUES WED THU FRI SAT SUN Cal Fat Pro Carbs

B ______
L ______
S ______
D ______

DAY 15: **MON TUES WED THU FRI SAT SUN** *Time* *Calories Burned*

Exercise ____________________

Water ____________ Steps ____________

Sleep ____________ Weight ____________

Stress Level 0 1 2 3 4 5 6 7 8 9 10 11

DAY 16: **MON TUES WED THU FRI SAT SUN** *Time* *Calories Burned*

Exercise ____________________

Water ____________ Steps ____________

Sleep ____________ Weight ____________

Stress Level 0 1 2 3 4 5 6 7 8 9 10 11

DAY 17: **MON TUES WED THU FRI SAT SUN** *Time* *Calories Burned*

Exercise ____________________

Water ____________ Steps ____________

Sleep ____________ Weight ____________

Stress Level 0 1 2 3 4 5 6 7 8 9 10 11

DAY 18: **MON TUES WED THU FRI SAT SUN** *Time* *Calories Burned*

Exercise ____________________

Water ____________ Steps ____________

Sleep ____________ Weight ____________

Stress Level 0 1 2 3 4 5 6 7 8 9 10 11

DAY 19: **MON TUES WED THU FRI SAT SUN** *Time* *Calories Burned*

Exercise ____________________

Water ____________ Steps ____________

Sleep ____________ Weight ____________

Stress Level 0 1 2 3 4 5 6 7 8 9 10 11

DAY 20: **MON TUES WED THU FRI SAT SUN** *Time* *Calories Burned*

Exercise ____________________

Water ____________ Steps ____________

Sleep ____________ Weight ____________

Stress Level 0 1 2 3 4 5 6 7 8 9 10 11

DAY 21: **MON TUES WED THU FRI SAT SUN** *Time* *Calories Burned*

Exercise ____________________

Water ____________ Steps ____________

Sleep ____________ Weight ____________

Stress Level 0 1 2 3 4 5 6 7 8 9 10 11

MEAL PLANNER * MONTH ______ YR ____

DAY 22: **MON TUES WED THU FRI SAT SUN** Cal Fat Pro Carbs

B ______
L ______
S ______
D ______

DAY 23: **MON TUES WED THU FRI SAT SUN** Cal Fat Pro Carbs

B ______
L ______
S ______
D ______

DAY 24: **MON TUES WED THU FRI SAT SUN** Cal Fat Pro Carbs

B ______
L ______
S ______
D ______

DAY 25: **MON TUES WED THU FRI SAT SUN** Cal Fat Pro Carbs

B ______
L ______
S ______
D ______

DAY 26: **MON TUES WED THU FRI SAT SUN** Cal Fat Pro Carbs

B ______
L ______
S ______
D ______

DAY 27: **MON TUES WED THU FRI SAT SUN** Cal Fat Pro Carbs

B ______
L ______
S ______
D ______

DAY 28: **MON TUES WED THU FRI SAT SUN** Cal Fat Pro Carbs

B ______
L ______
S ______
D ______

DAY 22: **MON TUES WED THU FRI SAT SUN** *Time* *Calories Burned*

Exercise ______

Water ______ Steps ______

Sleep ______ Weight ______

Stress Level 0 1 2 3 4 5 6 7 8 9 10 11

DAY 23: **MON TUES WED THU FRI SAT SUN** *Time* *Calories Burned*

Exercise ______

Water ______ Steps ______

Sleep ______ Weight ______

Stress Level 0 1 2 3 4 5 6 7 8 9 10 11

DAY 24: **MON TUES WED THU FRI SAT SUN** *Time* *Calories Burned*

Exercise ______

Water ______ Steps ______

Sleep ______ Weight ______

Stress Level 0 1 2 3 4 5 6 7 8 9 10 11

DAY 25: **MON TUES WED THU FRI SAT SUN** *Time* *Calories Burned*

Exercise ______

Water ______ Steps ______

Sleep ______ Weight ______

Stress Level 0 1 2 3 4 5 6 7 8 9 10 11

DAY 26: **MON TUES WED THU FRI SAT SUN** *Time* *Calories Burned*

Exercise ______

Water ______ Steps ______

Sleep ______ Weight ______

Stress Level 0 1 2 3 4 5 6 7 8 9 10 11

DAY 27: **MON TUES WED THU FRI SAT SUN** *Time* *Calories Burned*

Exercise ______

Water ______ Steps ______

Sleep ______ Weight ______

Stress Level 0 1 2 3 4 5 6 7 8 9 10 11

DAY 28: **MON TUES WED THU FRI SAT SUN** *Time* *Calories Burned*

Exercise ______

Water ______ Steps ______

Sleep ______ Weight ______

Stress Level 0 1 2 3 4 5 6 7 8 9 10 11

MEAL PLANNER * MONTH ________ YR ____

DAY 29: **MON TUES WED THU FRI SAT SUN** Cal Fat Pro Carbs

B ____________________

L ____________________

S ____________________

D ____________________

DAY 30: **MON TUES WED THU FRI SAT SUN** Cal Fat Pro Carbs

B ____________________

L ____________________

S ____________________

D ____________________

DAY 31: **MON TUES WED THU FRI SAT SUN** Cal Fat Pro Carbs

B ____________________

L ____________________

S ____________________

D ____________________

GOALS

Achieved Y N

1. ____________________ ☐ ☐
2. ____________________ ☐ ☐
3. ____________________ ☐ ☐
4. ____________________ ☐ ☐
5. ____________________ ☐ ☐

End of Month Results

Weight *Blood Pressure* *Resting Heart Rate*

DAY 29: **MON TUES WED THU FRI SAT SUN** *Time* *Calories Burned*

Exercise ______________________________

Water ____________ Steps ____________

Sleep ____________ Weight ____________

Stress Level 0 1 2 3 4 5 6 7 8 9 10 11

DAY 30: **MON TUES WED THU FRI SAT SUN** *Time* *Calories Burned*

Exercise ______________________________

Water ____________ Steps ____________

Sleep ____________ Weight ____________

Stress Level 0 1 2 3 4 5 6 7 8 9 10 11

DAY 31: **MON TUES WED THU FRI SAT SUN** *Time* *Calories Burned*

Exercise ______________________________

Water ____________ Steps ____________

Sleep ____________ Weight ____________

Stress Level 0 1 2 3 4 5 6 7 8 9 10 11

STRESSORS

	Resolved Y	Resolved N
1. ______________	☐	☐
2. ______________	☐	☐
3. ______________	☐	☐
4. ______________	☐	☐
5. ______________	☐	☐

of Successful Days

Count all the days this month you achieved your own health goals.

Exercise ◯ Water ◯ Steps ◯ Sleep ◯ Weight ◯

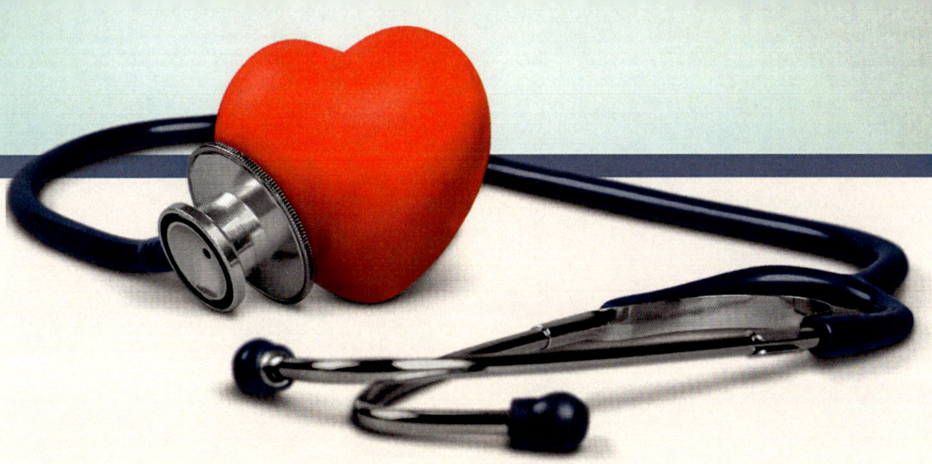

2. HEART

Arteries, Valve, Cholesterol

Without your heart, you can't live. We can live without every other part of our body, except our heart. Life ends when the heartbeat stops. It's very important to know that emotions affect your heart health. Too much stress is felt by your heart. It responds to that stress by beating faster. Emotional eating overloads your system. Poor eating clogs up our arteries. Our arteries are the highways away from the heart. Veins bring the blood back to the heart. What you send out comes back to you.

Set some goals for the month, and at the end, we will reflect on your progress. You can track your meals, exercise, appointments, and weight goals. Set some spiritual goals too.

GOALS

1. ______________________________
2. ______________________________
3. ______________________________
4. ______________________________
5. ______________________________

"Above all else, guard your heart,
for everything you do flows from it."
Proverbs 4:23

Monthly Affirmation:

"I am aware of my emotions."

Exercise: *React to only 50% of the triggers that once so easily beset you. Instead count to 20.*

FOODS to Improve Heart Health:

- **Beans:** Black Beans
- **Fat:** Olive Oil
- **Fruit:** Orange, Apple, Pear, Carrots
- **Herb:** Sage, Oregano, Rosemary, Thyme
- **Protein:** Farm-raised Salmon
- **Nuts:** Walnuts, Pecans, Almonds, Macadamia Nut, Hazelnuts
- **Root:** Beet, Celery
- **Vegetables:** Swiss Chard, Broccoli, Cabbage, Peppers
- Vitamins: Coenzyme Q10, Magnesium

JUICE to Improve Heart Health:

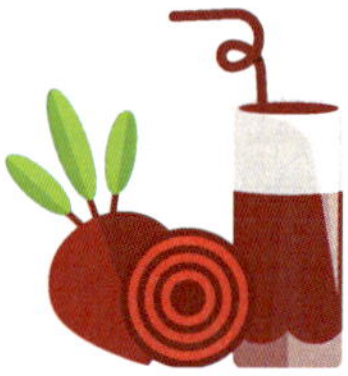

Beet
Celery
Orange

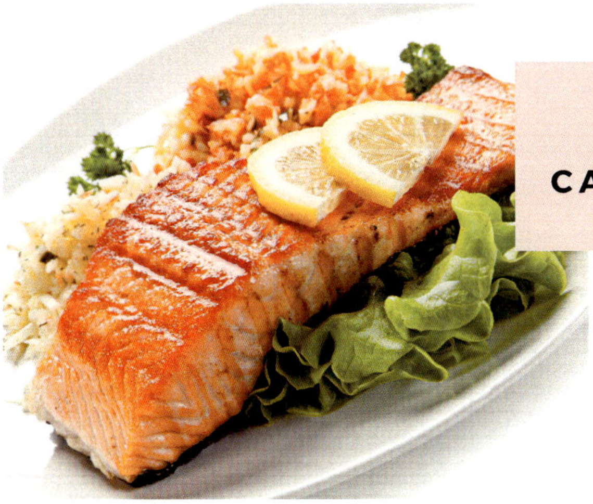

SALMON W/ CARAMELIZED PEARS

YIELDS 2 SERVINGS

PREP TIME: 30 MINS

2 - Salmon Fillets
1 - cup of Jasmine Rice
1/2 - cup chopped onion
1/2 - cup of water
1/2 - cup of chopped pears
3 tbsp - butter
3 tbsp - sugar
1 - tbsp of Olive Oil
1 - dash of salt
1 - dash of ground pepper

Optional:
Rosemary, Sage, Thyme

DIRECTIONS:

- Heat over to Broil Setting (425 degrees)
- Coat Salmon with olive oil, salt, pepper
- Add Salmon Skin-side down in baking dish
- Broil for 15 - 20 minutes
- In medium sauce pan add 1 cup of Jasmine rice to 1 1/4 cup of water. Boil and cover.
- Cook for 15 minutes or when water is gone
- In another saucepan, heat to Medium
- Add water and butter to melt
- Add onions, pears, and sugar to pan
- Cook for 10 minutes or until golden
- Add herbs to rice and serve
- Serve Pears/Onions on Salmon fillets

Medical Appointments

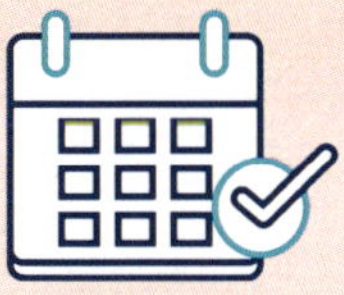

Date/Time	Office

MEAL PLANNER * MONTH ______ YR ____

DAY 1: **MON TUES WED THU FRI SAT SUN** Cal Fat Pro Carbs

B ____
L ____
S ____
D ____

DAY 2: **MON TUES WED THU FRI SAT SUN** Cal Fat Pro Carbs

B ____
L ____
S ____
D ____

DAY 3: **MON TUES WED THU FRI SAT SUN** Cal Fat Pro Carbs

B ____
L ____
S ____
D ____

DAY 4: **MON TUES WED THU FRI SAT SUN** Cal Fat Pro Carbs

B ____
L ____
S ____
D ____

DAY 5: **MON TUES WED THU FRI SAT SUN** Cal Fat Pro Carbs

B ____
L ____
S ____
D ____

DAY 6: **MON TUES WED THU FRI SAT SUN** Cal Fat Pro Carbs

B ____
L ____
S ____
D ____

DAY 7: **MON TUES WED THU FRI SAT SUN** Cal Fat Pro Carbs

B ____
L ____
S ____
D ____

DAY 1: **MON TUES WED THU FRI SAT SUN** *Time* *Calories Burned*

Exercise ________________________________

Water ______________ Steps ______________

Sleep ______________ Weight ______________

Stress Level 0 1 2 3 4 5 6 7 8 9 10 11

DAY 2: **MON TUES WED THU FRI SAT SUN** *Time* *Calories Burned*

Exercise ________________________________

Water ______________ Steps ______________

Sleep ______________ Weight ______________

Stress Level 0 1 2 3 4 5 6 7 8 9 10 11

DAY 3: **MON TUES WED THU FRI SAT SUN** *Time* *Calories Burned*

Exercise ________________________________

Water ______________ Steps ______________

Sleep ______________ Weight ______________

Stress Level 0 1 2 3 4 5 6 7 8 9 10 11

DAY 4: **MON TUES WED THU FRI SAT SUN** *Time* *Calories Burned*

Exercise ________________________________

Water ______________ Steps ______________

Sleep ______________ Weight ______________

Stress Level 0 1 2 3 4 5 6 7 8 9 10 11

DAY 5: **MON TUES WED THU FRI SAT SUN** *Time* *Calories Burned*

Exercise ________________________________

Water ______________ Steps ______________

Sleep ______________ Weight ______________

Stress Level 0 1 2 3 4 5 6 7 8 9 10 11

DAY 6: **MON TUES WED THU FRI SAT SUN** *Time* *Calories Burned*

Exercise ________________________________

Water ______________ Steps ______________

Sleep ______________ Weight ______________

Stress Level 0 1 2 3 4 5 6 7 8 9 10 11

DAY 7: **MON TUES WED THU FRI SAT SUN** *Time* *Calories Burned*

Exercise ________________________________

Water ______________ Steps ______________

Sleep ______________ Weight ______________

Stress Level 0 1 2 3 4 5 6 7 8 9 10 11

MEAL PLANNER * MONTH ________ YR ____

DAY 8: **MON TUES WED THU FRI SAT SUN** Cal Fat Pro Carbs

B ____________________

L ____________________

S ____________________

D ____________________

DAY 9: **MON TUES WED THU FRI SAT SUN** Cal Fat Pro Carbs

B ____________________

L ____________________

S ____________________

D ____________________

DAY 10: **MON TUES WED THU FRI SAT SUN** Cal Fat Pro Carbs

B ____________________

L ____________________

S ____________________

D ____________________

DAY 11: **MON TUES WED THU FRI SAT SUN** Cal Fat Pro Carbs

B ____________________

L ____________________

S ____________________

D ____________________

DAY 12: **MON TUES WED THU FRI SAT SUN** Cal Fat Pro Carbs

B ____________________

L ____________________

S ____________________

D ____________________

DAY 13: **MON TUES WED THU FRI SAT SUN** Cal Fat Pro Carbs

B ____________________

L ____________________

S ____________________

D ____________________

DAY 14: **MON TUES WED THU FRI SAT SUN** Cal Fat Pro Carbs

B ____________________

L ____________________

S ____________________

D ____________________

DAY 8: **MON TUES WED THU FRI SAT SUN** *Time* *Calories Burned*

Exercise ______________________________

Water ____________ Steps ____________

Sleep ____________ Weight ____________

Stress Level 0 1 2 3 4 5 6 7 8 9 10 11

DAY 9: **MON TUES WED THU FRI SAT SUN** *Time* *Calories Burned*

Exercise ______________________________

Water ____________ Steps ____________

Sleep ____________ Weight ____________

Stress Level 0 1 2 3 4 5 6 7 8 9 10 11

DAY 10: **MON TUES WED THU FRI SAT SUN** *Time* *Calories Burned*

Exercise ______________________________

Water ____________ Steps ____________

Sleep ____________ Weight ____________

Stress Level 0 1 2 3 4 5 6 7 8 9 10 11

DAY 11: **MON TUES WED THU FRI SAT SUN** *Time* *Calories Burned*

Exercise ______________________________

Water ____________ Steps ____________

Sleep ____________ Weight ____________

Stress Level 0 1 2 3 4 5 6 7 8 9 10 11

DAY 12: **MON TUES WED THU FRI SAT SUN** *Time* *Calories Burned*

Exercise ______________________________

Water ____________ Steps ____________

Sleep ____________ Weight ____________

Stress Level 0 1 2 3 4 5 6 7 8 9 10 11

DAY 13: **MON TUES WED THU FRI SAT SUN** *Time* *Calories Burned*

Exercise ______________________________

Water ____________ Steps ____________

Sleep ____________ Weight ____________

Stress Level 0 1 2 3 4 5 6 7 8 9 10 11

DAY 14: **MON TUES WED THU FRI SAT SUN** *Time* *Calories Burned*

Exercise ______________________________

Water ____________ Steps ____________

Sleep ____________ Weight ____________

Stress Level 0 1 2 3 4 5 6 7 8 9 10 11

MEAL PLANNER * MONTH ______ YR ______

DAY 15: **MON TUES WED THU FRI SAT SUN** Cal Fat Pro Carbs

B ____

L ____

S ____

D ____

DAY 16: **MON TUES WED THU FRI SAT SUN** Cal Fat Pro Carbs

B ____

L ____

S ____

D ____

DAY 17: **MON TUES WED THU FRI SAT SUN** Cal Fat Pro Carbs

B ____

L ____

S ____

D ____

DAY 18: **MON TUES WED THU FRI SAT SUN** Cal Fat Pro Carbs

B ____

L ____

S ____

D ____

DAY 19: **MON TUES WED THU FRI SAT SUN** Cal Fat Pro Carbs

B ____

L ____

S ____

D ____

DAY 20: **MON TUES WED THU FRI SAT SUN** Cal Fat Pro Carbs

B ____

L ____

S ____

D ____

DAY 21: **MON TUES WED THU FRI SAT SUN** Cal Fat Pro Carbs

B ____

L ____

S ____

D ____

DAY 15: **MON TUES WED THU FRI SAT SUN** *Time* *Calories Burned*

Exercise

Water Steps

Sleep Weight

Stress Level 0 1 2 3 4 5 6 7 8 9 10 11

DAY 16: **MON TUES WED THU FRI SAT SUN** *Time* *Calories Burned*

Exercise

Water Steps

Sleep Weight

Stress Level 0 1 2 3 4 5 6 7 8 9 10 11

DAY 17: **MON TUES WED THU FRI SAT SUN** *Time* *Calories Burned*

Exercise

Water Steps

Sleep Weight

Stress Level 0 1 2 3 4 5 6 7 8 9 10 11

DAY 18: **MON TUES WED THU FRI SAT SUN** *Time* *Calories Burned*

Exercise

Water Steps

Sleep Weight

Stress Level 0 1 2 3 4 5 6 7 8 9 10 11

DAY 19: **MON TUES WED THU FRI SAT SUN** *Time* *Calories Burned*

Exercise

Water Steps

Sleep Weight

Stress Level 0 1 2 3 4 5 6 7 8 9 10 11

DAY 20: **MON TUES WED THU FRI SAT SUN** *Time* *Calories Burned*

Exercise

Water Steps

Sleep Weight

Stress Level 0 1 2 3 4 5 6 7 8 9 10 11

DAY 21: **MON TUES WED THU FRI SAT SUN** *Time* *Calories Burned*

Exercise

Water Steps

Sleep Weight

Stress Level 0 1 2 3 4 5 6 7 8 9 10 11

MEAL PLANNER * MONTH ________ YR ____

DAY 22: MON TUES WED THU FRI SAT SUN Cal Fat Pro Carbs

B ____________________

L ____________________

S ____________________

D ____________________

DAY 23: MON TUES WED THU FRI SAT SUN Cal Fat Pro Carbs

B ____________________

L ____________________

S ____________________

D ____________________

DAY 24: MON TUES WED THU FRI SAT SUN Cal Fat Pro Carbs

B ____________________

L ____________________

S ____________________

D ____________________

DAY 25: MON TUES WED THU FRI SAT SUN Cal Fat Pro Carbs

B ____________________

L ____________________

S ____________________

D ____________________

DAY 26: MON TUES WED THU FRI SAT SUN Cal Fat Pro Carbs

B ____________________

L ____________________

S ____________________

D ____________________

DAY 27: MON TUES WED THU FRI SAT SUN Cal Fat Pro Carbs

B ____________________

L ____________________

S ____________________

D ____________________

DAY 28: MON TUES WED THU FRI SAT SUN Cal Fat Pro Carbs

B ____________________

L ____________________

S ____________________

D ____________________

DAY 22: **MON TUES WED THU FRI SAT SUN** *Time* *Calories Burned*

Exercise ______

Water ______ Steps ______

Sleep ______ Weight ______

Stress Level 0 1 2 3 4 5 6 7 8 9 10 11

DAY 23: **MON TUES WED THU FRI SAT SUN** *Time* *Calories Burned*

Exercise ______

Water ______ Steps ______

Sleep ______ Weight ______

Stress Level 0 1 2 3 4 5 6 7 8 9 10 11

DAY 24: **MON TUES WED THU FRI SAT SUN** *Time* *Calories Burned*

Exercise ______

Water ______ Steps ______

Sleep ______ Weight ______

Stress Level 0 1 2 3 4 5 6 7 8 9 10 11

DAY 25: **MON TUES WED THU FRI SAT SUN** *Time* *Calories Burned*

Exercise ______

Water ______ Steps ______

Sleep ______ Weight ______

Stress Level 0 1 2 3 4 5 6 7 8 9 10 11

DAY 26: **MON TUES WED THU FRI SAT SUN** *Time* *Calories Burned*

Exercise ______

Water ______ Steps ______

Sleep ______ Weight ______

Stress Level 0 1 2 3 4 5 6 7 8 9 10 11

DAY 27: **MON TUES WED THU FRI SAT SUN** *Time* *Calories Burned*

Exercise ______

Water ______ Steps ______

Sleep ______ Weight ______

Stress Level 0 1 2 3 4 5 6 7 8 9 10 11

DAY 28: **MON TUES WED THU FRI SAT SUN** *Time* *Calories Burned*

Exercise ______

Water ______ Steps ______

Sleep ______ Weight ______

Stress Level 0 1 2 3 4 5 6 7 8 9 10 11

MEAL PLANNER * MONTH ______ YR ____

DAY 29: **MON TUES WED THU FRI SAT SUN** Cal Fat Pro Carbs

B ______

L ______

S ______

D ______

DAY 30: **MON TUES WED THU FRI SAT SUN** Cal Fat Pro Carbs

B ______

L ______

S ______

D ______

DAY 31: **MON TUES WED THU FRI SAT SUN** Cal Fat Pro Carbs

B ______

L ______

S ______

D ______

GOALS

Achieved
Y N

1. ______ ☐ ☐
2. ______ ☐ ☐
3. ______ ☐ ☐
4. ______ ☐ ☐
5. ______ ☐ ☐

End of Month Results

Weight

Blood Pressure

Resting Heart Rate

DAY 29: **MON TUES WED THU FRI SAT SUN** *Time* *Calories Burned*

Exercise ____________________

Water ____________ Steps ____________

Sleep ____________ Weight ____________

Stress Level 0 1 2 3 4 5 6 7 8 9 10 11

DAY 30: **MON TUES WED THU FRI SAT SUN** *Time* *Calories Burned*

Exercise ____________________

Water ____________ Steps ____________

Sleep ____________ Weight ____________

Stress Level 0 1 2 3 4 5 6 7 8 9 10 11

DAY 31: **MON TUES WED THU FRI SAT SUN** *Time* *Calories Burned*

Exercise ____________________

Water ____________ Steps ____________

Sleep ____________ Weight ____________

Stress Level 0 1 2 3 4 5 6 7 8 9 10 11

STRESSORS

	Resolved Y	Resolved N
1. ____________________	☐	☐
2. ____________________	☐	☐
3. ____________________	☐	☐
4. ____________________	☐	☐
5. ____________________	☐	☐

of Successful Days

Count all the days this month you achieved your own health goals.

Exercise ◯ Water ◯ Steps ◯ Sleep ◯ Weight ◯

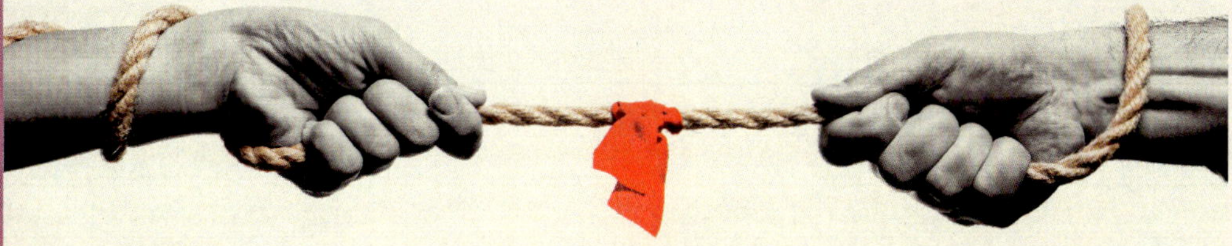

3. URINARY

Kidney, Bladder, Urethra, Ureters, Renal Pelvis

Fear stops us from Letting Go of things we should. It's very interesting that the area associated with letting things go is in our urinary system. We drink and we eliminate. If we hold onto it, our bodies become toxic. This liquid carries with it toxins, nutrients we can't absorb, and many other things we don't need. Anger is a toxic force that we hold onto. When we forgive, we eliminate anger, rage, and hurt from our bodies.

Set some goals for the month, and at the end, we will reflect on your progress. You can track your meals, exercise, appointments, and weight goals. Set some spiritual goals too.

GOALS

1. ______________________________
2. ______________________________
3. ______________________________
4. ______________________________
5. ______________________________

"Be angry and do not sin; do not let the sun go down on your anger, and give no opportunity to the devil."
Ephesians 4:26-27

Monthly Affirmation:

"I am letting go of what no longer serves me."

Exercise: *Every day, write down 5 things that made you unhappy. At the end of the day, throw it away.*

FOODS to Improve Urinary Health:

- **Beans:** Green Beans
- **Fat:** Olive Oil, Egg Whites
- **Fruit:** Blueberries, Apples, Red Grapes, Cranberries
- **Herb:** Beetroot, Parsley, Ginger
- **Protein:** Sea-Bass, Skinless Chicken
- **Nuts:** Macadamia Nut
- **Root:** Sweet Potato, Radish, Turnip
- **Vegetables:** Cauliflower, Cabbage, Bell Pepper, Shiitake
- Vitamins: B2, B6, B12, Folic Acid, Magnesium, Niacin

JUICE to Improve Urinary Health:

Cranberry Ginger

Contact Vandene:
for Local South Florida Delivery
ordersmavis@gmail.com

M.A.V.I.S
Health Drinks

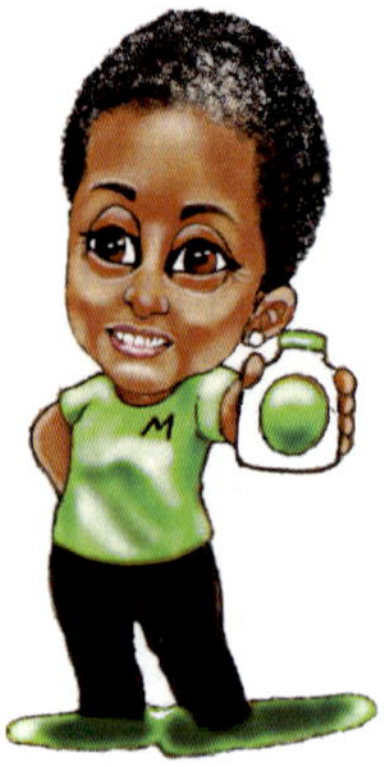

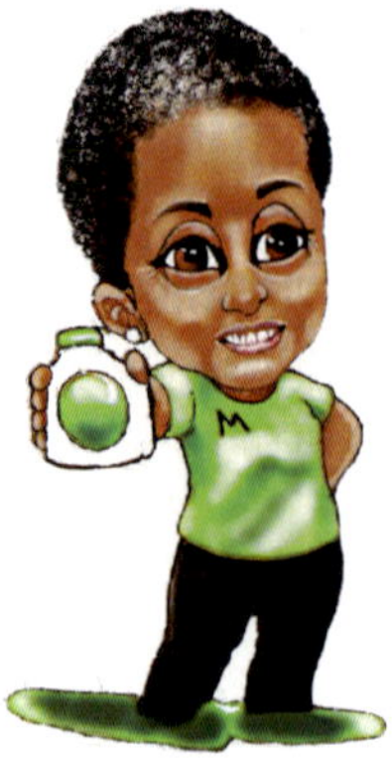

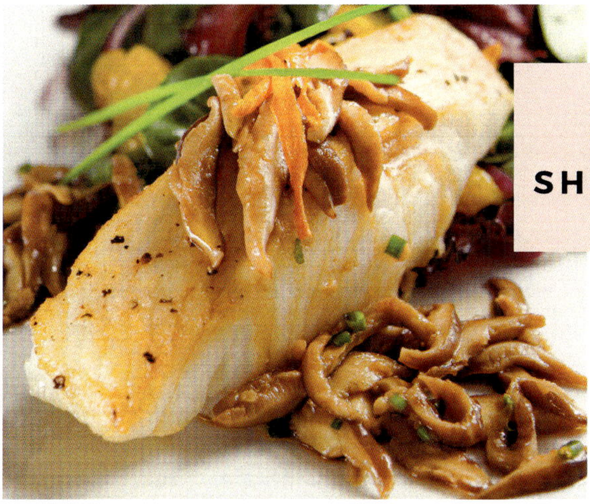

SEA BASS W/ SHIITAKE MUSHROOMS

YIELDS 2 SERVINGS

TOTAL TIME: 15 MINS

2 - Skinless Bass Fillets
1 - cup of Shiitake mushroom caps
1/2 - cup Scallions, chopped
1/4 - cup of water
1 - tsp of fresh ground ginger
2 tbsp - low-sodium soy sauce
1 tsp - Minced Garlic
1 - tbsp of Olive Oil
1 - tsp of Lemon juice
1 - dash of salt
1 - dash of ground pepper

Optional:
Rosemary, Sage, Thyme

DIRECTIONS:

- Heat oil in a nonstick pan to Medium-High
- Season Sea Bass with salt and pepper
- Add fish to pain, and cook for 3 minutes
- Turn over and cook again for 3 minutes
- When flaky, remove and cover in a plate
- In same pan, add Shiitake and soy sauce, and Sauté for 2 minutes
- Add Ginger, Garlic, Scallions
- Add Lemon Juice, water
- Add Rosemary, Sage or Thyme (optional)
- Sauté for 2 more minutes
- Serve fish on a bed of Shiitake mushrooms

Medical Appointments

Date/Time	Office

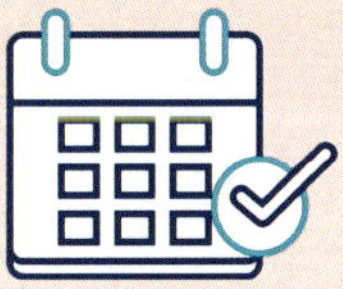

MEAL PLANNER * MONTH ______ YR ____

DAY 1: **MON TUES WED THU FRI SAT SUN** Cal Fat Pro Carbs

B ______

L ______

S ______

D ______

DAY 2: **MON TUES WED THU FRI SAT SUN** Cal Fat Pro Carbs

B ______

L ______

S ______

D ______

DAY 3: **MON TUES WED THU FRI SAT SUN** Cal Fat Pro Carbs

B ______

L ______

S ______

D ______

DAY 4: **MON TUES WED THU FRI SAT SUN** Cal Fat Pro Carbs

B ______

L ______

S ______

D ______

DAY 5: **MON TUES WED THU FRI SAT SUN** Cal Fat Pro Carbs

B ______

L ______

S ______

D ______

DAY 6: **MON TUES WED THU FRI SAT SUN** Cal Fat Pro Carbs

B ______

L ______

S ______

D ______

DAY 7: **MON TUES WED THU FRI SAT SUN** Cal Fat Pro Carbs

B ______

L ______

S ______

D ______

DAY 1: **MON TUES WED THU FRI SAT SUN** *Time* *Calories Burned*

Exercise ______________________________

Water ____________ Steps ____________

Sleep ____________ Weight ____________

Stress Level 0 1 2 3 4 5 6 7 8 9 10 11

DAY 2: **MON TUES WED THU FRI SAT SUN** *Time* *Calories Burned*

Exercise ______________________________

Water ____________ Steps ____________

Sleep ____________ Weight ____________

Stress Level 0 1 2 3 4 5 6 7 8 9 10 11

DAY 3: **MON TUES WED THU FRI SAT SUN** *Time* *Calories Burned*

Exercise ______________________________

Water ____________ Steps ____________

Sleep ____________ Weight ____________

Stress Level 0 1 2 3 4 5 6 7 8 9 10 11

DAY 4: **MON TUES WED THU FRI SAT SUN** *Time* *Calories Burned*

Exercise ______________________________

Water ____________ Steps ____________

Sleep ____________ Weight ____________

Stress Level 0 1 2 3 4 5 6 7 8 9 10 11

DAY 5: **MON TUES WED THU FRI SAT SUN** *Time* *Calories Burned*

Exercise ______________________________

Water ____________ Steps ____________

Sleep ____________ Weight ____________

Stress Level 0 1 2 3 4 5 6 7 8 9 10 11

DAY 6: **MON TUES WED THU FRI SAT SUN** *Time* *Calories Burned*

Exercise ______________________________

Water ____________ Steps ____________

Sleep ____________ Weight ____________

Stress Level 0 1 2 3 4 5 6 7 8 9 10 11

DAY 7: **MON TUES WED THU FRI SAT SUN** *Time* *Calories Burned*

Exercise ______________________________

Water ____________ Steps ____________

Sleep ____________ Weight ____________

Stress Level 0 1 2 3 4 5 6 7 8 9 10 11

MEAL PLANNER * MONTH ________ YR ______

DAY 8: **MON TUES WED THU FRI SAT SUN** Cal Fat Pro Carbs

B ____

L ____

S ____

D ____

DAY 9: **MON TUES WED THU FRI SAT SUN** Cal Fat Pro Carbs

B ____

L ____

S ____

D ____

DAY 10: **MON TUES WED THU FRI SAT SUN** Cal Fat Pro Carbs

B ____

L ____

S ____

D ____

DAY 11: **MON TUES WED THU FRI SAT SUN** Cal Fat Pro Carbs

B ____

L ____

S ____

D ____

DAY 12: **MON TUES WED THU FRI SAT SUN** Cal Fat Pro Carbs

B ____

L ____

S ____

D ____

DAY 13: **MON TUES WED THU FRI SAT SUN** Cal Fat Pro Carbs

B ____

L ____

S ____

D ____

DAY 14: **MON TUES WED THU FRI SAT SUN** Cal Fat Pro Carbs

B ____

L ____

S ____

D ____

DAY 8: **MON TUES WED THU FRI SAT SUN** *Time* *Calories Burned*

Exercise ______
Water ______ Steps ______
Sleep ______ Weight ______
Stress Level 0 1 2 3 4 5 6 7 8 9 10 11

DAY 9: **MON TUES WED THU FRI SAT SUN** *Time* *Calories Burned*

Exercise ______
Water ______ Steps ______
Sleep ______ Weight ______
Stress Level 0 1 2 3 4 5 6 7 8 9 10 11

DAY 10: **MON TUES WED THU FRI SAT SUN** *Time* *Calories Burned*

Exercise ______
Water ______ Steps ______
Sleep ______ Weight ______
Stress Level 0 1 2 3 4 5 6 7 8 9 10 11

DAY 11: **MON TUES WED THU FRI SAT SUN** *Time* *Calories Burned*

Exercise ______
Water ______ Steps ______
Sleep ______ Weight ______
Stress Level 0 1 2 3 4 5 6 7 8 9 10 11

DAY 12: **MON TUES WED THU FRI SAT SUN** *Time* *Calories Burned*

Exercise ______
Water ______ Steps ______
Sleep ______ Weight ______
Stress Level 0 1 2 3 4 5 6 7 8 9 10 11

DAY 13: **MON TUES WED THU FRI SAT SUN** *Time* *Calories Burned*

Exercise ______
Water ______ Steps ______
Sleep ______ Weight ______
Stress Level 0 1 2 3 4 5 6 7 8 9 10 11

DAY 14: **MON TUES WED THU FRI SAT SUN** *Time* *Calories Burned*

Exercise ______
Water ______ Steps ______
Sleep ______ Weight ______
Stress Level 0 1 2 3 4 5 6 7 8 9 10 11

MEAL PLANNER * MONTH ________ YR ______

DAY 15: **MON TUES WED THU FRI SAT SUN** Cal Fat Pro Carbs

B ______

L ______

S ______

D ______

DAY 16: **MON TUES WED THU FRI SAT SUN** Cal Fat Pro Carbs

B ______

L ______

S ______

D ______

DAY 17: **MON TUES WED THU FRI SAT SUN** Cal Fat Pro Carbs

B ______

L ______

S ______

D ______

DAY 18: **MON TUES WED THU FRI SAT SUN** Cal Fat Pro Carbs

B ______

L ______

S ______

D ______

DAY 19: **MON TUES WED THU FRI SAT SUN** Cal Fat Pro Carbs

B ______

L ______

S ______

D ______

DAY 20: **MON TUES WED THU FRI SAT SUN** Cal Fat Pro Carbs

B ______

L ______

S ______

D ______

DAY 21: **MON TUES WED THU FRI SAT SUN** Cal Fat Pro Carbs

B ______

L ______

S ______

D ______

DAY 15: **MON TUES WED THU FRI SAT SUN** *Time* *Calories Burned*

Exercise ____________________

Water ____________ Steps ____________

Sleep ____________ Weight ____________

Stress Level 0 1 2 3 4 5 6 7 8 9 10 11

DAY 16: **MON TUES WED THU FRI SAT SUN** *Time* *Calories Burned*

Exercise ____________________

Water ____________ Steps ____________

Sleep ____________ Weight ____________

Stress Level 0 1 2 3 4 5 6 7 8 9 10 11

DAY 17: **MON TUES WED THU FRI SAT SUN** *Time* *Calories Burned*

Exercise ____________________

Water ____________ Steps ____________

Sleep ____________ Weight ____________

Stress Level 0 1 2 3 4 5 6 7 8 9 10 11

DAY 18: **MON TUES WED THU FRI SAT SUN** *Time* *Calories Burned*

Exercise ____________________

Water ____________ Steps ____________

Sleep ____________ Weight ____________

Stress Level 0 1 2 3 4 5 6 7 8 9 10 11

DAY 19: **MON TUES WED THU FRI SAT SUN** *Time* *Calories Burned*

Exercise ____________________

Water ____________ Steps ____________

Sleep ____________ Weight ____________

Stress Level 0 1 2 3 4 5 6 7 8 9 10 11

DAY 20: **MON TUES WED THU FRI SAT SUN** *Time* *Calories Burned*

Exercise ____________________

Water ____________ Steps ____________

Sleep ____________ Weight ____________

Stress Level 0 1 2 3 4 5 6 7 8 9 10 11

DAY 21: **MON TUES WED THU FRI SAT SUN** *Time* *Calories Burned*

Exercise ____________________

Water ____________ Steps ____________

Sleep ____________ Weight ____________

Stress Level 0 1 2 3 4 5 6 7 8 9 10 11

MEAL PLANNER * MONTH ________ YR ____

DAY 22: MON TUES WED THU FRI SAT SUN Cal Fat Pro Carbs

B ____
L ____
S ____
D ____

DAY 23: MON TUES WED THU FRI SAT SUN Cal Fat Pro Carbs

B ____
L ____
S ____
D ____

DAY 24: MON TUES WED THU FRI SAT SUN Cal Fat Pro Carbs

B ____
L ____
S ____
D ____

DAY 25: MON TUES WED THU FRI SAT SUN Cal Fat Pro Carbs

B ____
L ____
S ____
D ____

DAY 26: MON TUES WED THU FRI SAT SUN Cal Fat Pro Carbs

B ____
L ____
S ____
D ____

DAY 27: MON TUES WED THU FRI SAT SUN Cal Fat Pro Carbs

B ____
L ____
S ____
D ____

DAY 28: MON TUES WED THU FRI SAT SUN Cal Fat Pro Carbs

B ____
L ____
S ____
D ____

DAY 22: **MON TUES WED THU FRI SAT SUN** *Time* *Calories Burned*

Exercise ______

Water ______ Steps ______

Sleep ______ Weight ______

Stress Level 0 1 2 3 4 5 6 7 8 9 10 11

DAY 23: **MON TUES WED THU FRI SAT SUN** *Time* *Calories Burned*

Exercise ______

Water ______ Steps ______

Sleep ______ Weight ______

Stress Level 0 1 2 3 4 5 6 7 8 9 10 11

DAY 24: **MON TUES WED THU FRI SAT SUN** *Time* *Calories Burned*

Exercise ______

Water ______ Steps ______

Sleep ______ Weight ______

Stress Level 0 1 2 3 4 5 6 7 8 9 10 11

DAY 25: **MON TUES WED THU FRI SAT SUN** *Time* *Calories Burned*

Exercise ______

Water ______ Steps ______

Sleep ______ Weight ______

Stress Level 0 1 2 3 4 5 6 7 8 9 10 11

DAY 26: **MON TUES WED THU FRI SAT SUN** *Time* *Calories Burned*

Exercise ______

Water ______ Steps ______

Sleep ______ Weight ______

Stress Level 0 1 2 3 4 5 6 7 8 9 10 11

DAY 27: **MON TUES WED THU FRI SAT SUN** *Time* *Calories Burned*

Exercise ______

Water ______ Steps ______

Sleep ______ Weight ______

Stress Level 0 1 2 3 4 5 6 7 8 9 10 11

DAY 28: **MON TUES WED THU FRI SAT SUN** *Time* *Calories Burned*

Exercise ______

Water ______ Steps ______

Sleep ______ Weight ______

Stress Level 0 1 2 3 4 5 6 7 8 9 10 11

MEAL PLANNER * MONTH ________ YR ____

DAY 29: **MON TUES WED THU FRI SAT SUN** Cal Fat Pro Carbs

B ______

L ______

S ______

D ______

DAY 30: **MON TUES WED THU FRI SAT SUN** Cal Fat Pro Carbs

B ______

L ______

S ______

D ______

DAY 31: **MON TUES WED THU FRI SAT SUN** Cal Fat Pro Carbs

B ______

L ______

S ______

D ______

GOALS

	Achieved Y	N
1. ______	☐	☐
2. ______	☐	☐
3. ______	☐	☐
4. ______	☐	☐
5. ______	☐	☐

End of Month Results

Weight

Blood Pressure

Resting Heart Rate

DAY 29: **MON TUES WED THU FRI SAT SUN** *Time* *Calories Burned*

Exercise ____________________

Water ____________ Steps ____________

Sleep ____________ Weight ____________

Stress Level 0 1 2 3 4 5 6 7 8 9 10 11

DAY 30: **MON TUES WED THU FRI SAT SUN** *Time* *Calories Burned*

Exercise ____________________

Water ____________ Steps ____________

Sleep ____________ Weight ____________

Stress Level 0 1 2 3 4 5 6 7 8 9 10 11

DAY 31: **MON TUES WED THU FRI SAT SUN** *Time* *Calories Burned*

Exercise ____________________

Water ____________ Steps ____________

Sleep ____________ Weight ____________

Stress Level 0 1 2 3 4 5 6 7 8 9 10 11

STRESSORS

	Resolved Y	Resolved N
1. ____________	☐	☐
2. ____________	☐	☐
3. ____________	☐	☐
4. ____________	☐	☐
5. ____________	☐	☐

of Successful Days

Count all the days this month you achieved your own health goals.

Exercise Water Steps Sleep Weight

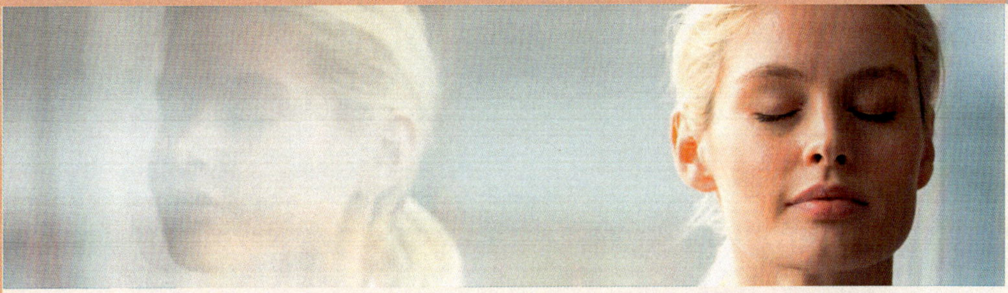

4. RESPIRATORY

Lungs, Trachea, Larynx

Lung problems are caused by "unshed tears". When we aren't able to express ourselves freely, we turn on ourselves, internally. This may not be intentional. It's just that we feel nobody cares enough. We become afraid to breathe, afraid to express, and afraid of abandonment. If we express ourselves too much, we'll be considered too needy. So, we pretend we don't need anything, and grieve in silence. Respiratory problems are caused by grief. How can we express our emotions without judgment?

Set some goals for the month, and at the end, we will reflect on your progress. You can track your meals, exercise, appointments, and weight goals. Set some spiritual goals too.

GOALS

1. ______________________________
2. ______________________________
3. ______________________________
4. ______________________________
5. ______________________________

> *"And God shall wipe away all tears from their eyes; and there shall be no more death, neither sorrow, nor crying, neither shall there be any more pain: for the former things are passed away."*
> *Revelations 21:4*

Monthly Affirmation:

"I am expressing myself in constructive ways."

Exercise: *This month, try to speak your truth in a constructive way. Find words that promote healing.*

FOODS to Improve Respiratory Health:

- **Beans:** Edamame, Lentils
- **Fat:** Olive Oil, Yogurt
- **Fruit:** Blueberries, Apples, Tomato
- **Herb:** Green Tea, Thyme
- **Protein:** Anchovies, Oysters
- **Nuts:** Brazil Nuts, Walnuts
- **Root:** Turmeric, Ginger, Garlic
- **Vegetables:** Butternut Squash, Peppers, Pumpkin, Red Cabbage, Swiss Chard
- Vitamins: Zinc, Selenium, Copper, B12, C, Potassium, Phosphorus, Calcium, Flaxseed

JUICE to Improve Respiratory Health:

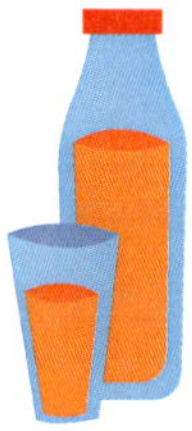

Turmeric
Cayenne
Ginger

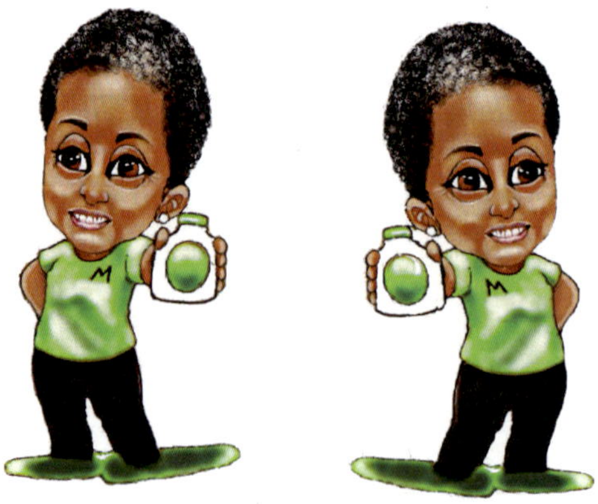

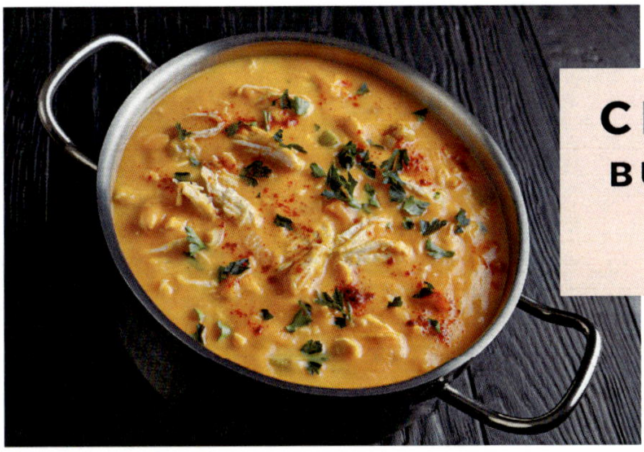

CHICKEN STEW/ BUTTERNUT SQUASH AND LENTILS

YIELDS 4 SERVINGS

TOTAL TIME: 30 MINS

2 - cups of Cooked Chicken
2 - cups of Butternut Squash Peeled and Diced
1 - cup chopped yellow onions
1 - cup of Red Lentils (rinsed)
1/2 - cup of Chopped Swiss Chard
2 - cups of water
1 - tsp of Curry powder
2 - tsp of Minced Ginger
1 - tbsp of Minced Garlic
1 - tbsp of Dried Thyme
2 - tbsp of Olive Oil
1 - tbsp of Lime juice
1 - dash of Kosher salt
1 - dash of ground pepper
1 - veggie boullion cube

DIRECTIONS:

- Heat Olive oil in a large stew pot to Medium
- Add Onion
- Add Garlic
- Add Ginger
- After 2 minutes, Add Butternut Squash
- After 2 minutes, Add curry powder
- Add salt and pepper
- Stir continuously for 1 minute
- Add lentils, boullion cube, and water
- Let it boil, then turn down to simmer
- Cook uncovered for 20 minutes
- Add Swiss Chard for 3 minutes
- Add cooked chicken and Thyme
- Add lime juice
- Cook for 2 minutes and serve

Medical Appointments

Date/Time Office

___

___

___

___

MEAL PLANNER * MONTH ______ YR ____

DAY 1: **MON TUES WED THU FRI SAT SUN** Cal Fat Pro Carbs

B ______

L ______

S ______

D ______

DAY 2: **MON TUES WED THU FRI SAT SUN** Cal Fat Pro Carbs

B ______

L ______

S ______

D ______

DAY 3: **MON TUES WED THU FRI SAT SUN** Cal Fat Pro Carbs

B ______

L ______

S ______

D ______

DAY 4: **MON TUES WED THU FRI SAT SUN** Cal Fat Pro Carbs

B ______

L ______

S ______

D ______

DAY 5: **MON TUES WED THU FRI SAT SUN** Cal Fat Pro Carbs

B ______

L ______

S ______

D ______

DAY 6: **MON TUES WED THU FRI SAT SUN** Cal Fat Pro Carbs

B ______

L ______

S ______

D ______

DAY 7: **MON TUES WED THU FRI SAT SUN** Cal Fat Pro Carbs

B ______

L ______

S ______

D ______

DAY 1: **MON TUES WED THU FRI SAT SUN** *Time* *Calories Burned*

Exercise ______________________________

Water ______________ Steps ______________

Sleep ______________ Weight ______________

Stress Level 0 1 2 3 4 5 6 7 8 9 10 11

DAY 2: **MON TUES WED THU FRI SAT SUN** *Time* *Calories Burned*

Exercise ______________________________

Water ______________ Steps ______________

Sleep ______________ Weight ______________

Stress Level 0 1 2 3 4 5 6 7 8 9 10 11

DAY 3: **MON TUES WED THU FRI SAT SUN** *Time* *Calories Burned*

Exercise ______________________________

Water ______________ Steps ______________

Sleep ______________ Weight ______________

Stress Level 0 1 2 3 4 5 6 7 8 9 10 11

DAY 4: **MON TUES WED THU FRI SAT SUN** *Time* *Calories Burned*

Exercise ______________________________

Water ______________ Steps ______________

Sleep ______________ Weight ______________

Stress Level 0 1 2 3 4 5 6 7 8 9 10 11

DAY 5: **MON TUES WED THU FRI SAT SUN** *Time* *Calories Burned*

Exercise ______________________________

Water ______________ Steps ______________

Sleep ______________ Weight ______________

Stress Level 0 1 2 3 4 5 6 7 8 9 10 11

DAY 6: **MON TUES WED THU FRI SAT SUN** *Time* *Calories Burned*

Exercise ______________________________

Water ______________ Steps ______________

Sleep ______________ Weight ______________

Stress Level 0 1 2 3 4 5 6 7 8 9 10 11

DAY 7: **MON TUES WED THU FRI SAT SUN** *Time* *Calories Burned*

Exercise ______________________________

Water ______________ Steps ______________

Sleep ______________ Weight ______________

Stress Level 0 1 2 3 4 5 6 7 8 9 10 11

DAY 8: **MON TUES WED THU FRI SAT SUN** Cal Fat Pro Carbs

B ____________________
L ____________________
S ____________________
D ____________________

DAY 9: **MON TUES WED THU FRI SAT SUN** Cal Fat Pro Carbs

B ____________________
L ____________________
S ____________________
D ____________________

DAY 10: **MON TUES WED THU FRI SAT SUN** Cal Fat Pro Carbs

B ____________________
L ____________________
S ____________________
D ____________________

DAY 11: **MON TUES WED THU FRI SAT SUN** Cal Fat Pro Carbs

B ____________________
L ____________________
S ____________________
D ____________________

DAY 12: **MON TUES WED THU FRI SAT SUN** Cal Fat Pro Carbs

B ____________________
L ____________________
S ____________________
D ____________________

DAY 13: **MON TUES WED THU FRI SAT SUN** Cal Fat Pro Carbs

B ____________________
L ____________________
S ____________________
D ____________________

DAY 14: **MON TUES WED THU FRI SAT SUN** Cal Fat Pro Carbs

B ____________________
L ____________________
S ____________________
D ____________________

DAY 8: **MON TUES WED THU FRI SAT SUN** *Time* *Calories Burned*

Exercise ________________________________

Water ______________ Steps ______________

Sleep ______________ Weight ______________

Stress Level 0 1 2 3 4 5 6 7 8 9 10 11

DAY 9: **MON TUES WED THU FRI SAT SUN** *Time* *Calories Burned*

Exercise ________________________________

Water ______________ Steps ______________

Sleep ______________ Weight ______________

Stress Level 0 1 2 3 4 5 6 7 8 9 10 11

DAY 10: **MON TUES WED THU FRI SAT SUN** *Time* *Calories Burned*

Exercise ________________________________

Water ______________ Steps ______________

Sleep ______________ Weight ______________

Stress Level 0 1 2 3 4 5 6 7 8 9 10 11

DAY 11: **MON TUES WED THU FRI SAT SUN** *Time* *Calories Burned*

Exercise ________________________________

Water ______________ Steps ______________

Sleep ______________ Weight ______________

Stress Level 0 1 2 3 4 5 6 7 8 9 10 11

DAY 12: **MON TUES WED THU FRI SAT SUN** *Time* *Calories Burned*

Exercise ________________________________

Water ______________ Steps ______________

Sleep ______________ Weight ______________

Stress Level 0 1 2 3 4 5 6 7 8 9 10 11

DAY 13: **MON TUES WED THU FRI SAT SUN** *Time* *Calories Burned*

Exercise ________________________________

Water ______________ Steps ______________

Sleep ______________ Weight ______________

Stress Level 0 1 2 3 4 5 6 7 8 9 10 11

DAY 14: **MON TUES WED THU FRI SAT SUN** *Time* *Calories Burned*

Exercise ________________________________

Water ______________ Steps ______________

Sleep ______________ Weight ______________

Stress Level 0 1 2 3 4 5 6 7 8 9 10 11

MEAL PLANNER * MONTH __________ YR ____

DAY 15: **MON TUES WED THU FRI SAT SUN** Cal Fat Pro Carbs

B ____________________

L ____________________

S ____________________

D ____________________

DAY 16: **MON TUES WED THU FRI SAT SUN** Cal Fat Pro Carbs

B ____________________

L ____________________

S ____________________

D ____________________

DAY 17: **MON TUES WED THU FRI SAT SUN** Cal Fat Pro Carbs

B ____________________

L ____________________

S ____________________

D ____________________

DAY 18: **MON TUES WED THU FRI SAT SUN** Cal Fat Pro Carbs

B ____________________

L ____________________

S ____________________

D ____________________

DAY 19: **MON TUES WED THU FRI SAT SUN** Cal Fat Pro Carbs

B ____________________

L ____________________

S ____________________

D ____________________

DAY 20: **MON TUES WED THU FRI SAT SUN** Cal Fat Pro Carbs

B ____________________

L ____________________

S ____________________

D ____________________

DAY 21: **MON TUES WED THU FRI SAT SUN** Cal Fat Pro Carbs

B ____________________

L ____________________

S ____________________

D ____________________

DAY 15: **MON TUES WED THU FRI SAT SUN** *Time* *Calories Burned*

Exercise ______

Water ______ Steps ______

Sleep ______ Weight ______

Stress Level 0 1 2 3 4 5 6 7 8 9 10 11

DAY 16: **MON TUES WED THU FRI SAT SUN** *Time* *Calories Burned*

Exercise ______

Water ______ Steps ______

Sleep ______ Weight ______

Stress Level 0 1 2 3 4 5 6 7 8 9 10 11

DAY 17: **MON TUES WED THU FRI SAT SUN** *Time* *Calories Burned*

Exercise ______

Water ______ Steps ______

Sleep ______ Weight ______

Stress Level 0 1 2 3 4 5 6 7 8 9 10 11

DAY 18: **MON TUES WED THU FRI SAT SUN** *Time* *Calories Burned*

Exercise ______

Water ______ Steps ______

Sleep ______ Weight ______

Stress Level 0 1 2 3 4 5 6 7 8 9 10 11

DAY 19: **MON TUES WED THU FRI SAT SUN** *Time* *Calories Burned*

Exercise ______

Water ______ Steps ______

Sleep ______ Weight ______

Stress Level 0 1 2 3 4 5 6 7 8 9 10 11

DAY 20: **MON TUES WED THU FRI SAT SUN** *Time* *Calories Burned*

Exercise ______

Water ______ Steps ______

Sleep ______ Weight ______

Stress Level 0 1 2 3 4 5 6 7 8 9 10 11

DAY 21: **MON TUES WED THU FRI SAT SUN** *Time* *Calories Burned*

Exercise ______

Water ______ Steps ______

Sleep ______ Weight ______

Stress Level 0 1 2 3 4 5 6 7 8 9 10 11

DAY 22: **MON TUES WED THU FRI SAT SUN** Cal Fat Pro Carbs

B ______
L ______
S ______
D ______

DAY 23: **MON TUES WED THU FRI SAT SUN** Cal Fat Pro Carbs

B ______
L ______
S ______
D ______

DAY 24: **MON TUES WED THU FRI SAT SUN** Cal Fat Pro Carbs

B ______
L ______
S ______
D ______

DAY 25: **MON TUES WED THU FRI SAT SUN** Cal Fat Pro Carbs

B ______
L ______
S ______
D ______

DAY 26: **MON TUES WED THU FRI SAT SUN** Cal Fat Pro Carbs

B ______
L ______
S ______
D ______

DAY 27: **MON TUES WED THU FRI SAT SUN** Cal Fat Pro Carbs

B ______
L ______
S ______
D ______

DAY 28: **MON TUES WED THU FRI SAT SUN** Cal Fat Pro Carbs

B ______
L ______
S ______
D ______

DAY 22: **MON TUES WED THU FRI SAT SUN** *Time* *Calories Burned*

Exercise ______________________________

Water ______________ Steps ______________

Sleep ______________ Weight ______________

Stress Level 0 1 2 3 4 5 6 7 8 9 10 11

DAY 23: **MON TUES WED THU FRI SAT SUN** *Time* *Calories Burned*

Exercise ______________________________

Water ______________ Steps ______________

Sleep ______________ Weight ______________

Stress Level 0 1 2 3 4 5 6 7 8 9 10 11

DAY 24: **MON TUES WED THU FRI SAT SUN** *Time* *Calories Burned*

Exercise ______________________________

Water ______________ Steps ______________

Sleep ______________ Weight ______________

Stress Level 0 1 2 3 4 5 6 7 8 9 10 11

DAY 25: **MON TUES WED THU FRI SAT SUN** *Time* *Calories Burned*

Exercise ______________________________

Water ______________ Steps ______________

Sleep ______________ Weight ______________

Stress Level 0 1 2 3 4 5 6 7 8 9 10 11

DAY 26: **MON TUES WED THU FRI SAT SUN** *Time* *Calories Burned*

Exercise ______________________________

Water ______________ Steps ______________

Sleep ______________ Weight ______________

Stress Level 0 1 2 3 4 5 6 7 8 9 10 11

DAY 27: **MON TUES WED THU FRI SAT SUN** *Time* *Calories Burned*

Exercise ______________________________

Water ______________ Steps ______________

Sleep ______________ Weight ______________

Stress Level 0 1 2 3 4 5 6 7 8 9 10 11

DAY 28: **MON TUES WED THU FRI SAT SUN** *Time* *Calories Burned*

Exercise ______________________________

Water ______________ Steps ______________

Sleep ______________ Weight ______________

Stress Level 0 1 2 3 4 5 6 7 8 9 10 11

MEAL PLANNER * MONTH ________ YR ______

DAY 29: MON TUES WED THU FRI SAT SUN Cal Fat Pro Carbs

B ____________________

L ____________________

S ____________________

D ____________________

DAY 30: MON TUES WED THU FRI SAT SUN Cal Fat Pro Carbs

B ____________________

L ____________________

S ____________________

D ____________________

DAY 31: MON TUES WED THU FRI SAT SUN Cal Fat Pro Carbs

B ____________________

L ____________________

S ____________________

D ____________________

GOALS

	Achieved Y	N
1. ____________________	☐	☐
2. ____________________	☐	☐
3. ____________________	☐	☐
4. ____________________	☐	☐
5. ____________________	☐	☐

End of Month Results

Weight

Blood Pressure

Resting Heart Rate

DAY 29: **MON TUES WED THU FRI SAT SUN** *Time* *Calories Burned*

Exercise ___

Water ___ Steps ___

Sleep ___ Weight ___

Stress Level 0 1 2 3 4 5 6 7 8 9 10 11

DAY 30: **MON TUES WED THU FRI SAT SUN** *Time* *Calories Burned*

Exercise ___

Water ___ Steps ___

Sleep ___ Weight ___

Stress Level 0 1 2 3 4 5 6 7 8 9 10 11

DAY 31: **MON TUES WED THU FRI SAT SUN** *Time* *Calories Burned*

Exercise ___

Water ___ Steps ___

Sleep ___ Weight ___

Stress Level 0 1 2 3 4 5 6 7 8 9 10 11

STRESSORS

Resolved

	Y	N
1. ___	☐	☐
2. ___	☐	☐
3. ___	☐	☐
4. ___	☐	☐
5. ___	☐	☐

of Successful Days

Count all the days this month you achieved your own health goals.

Exercise ◯ Water ◯ Steps ◯ Sleep ◯ Weight ◯

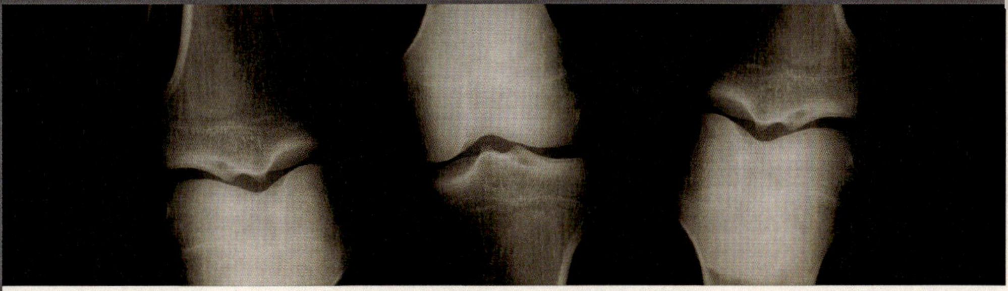

5. BONES

Skeletal, Arthritis, Osteoporosis

The skeletal structure of our bodies are the framework that everything else is built on. Without our bones, we couldn't walk, stand, lie down, or move our arms. It's the foundation of every other system. When we have bone issues, we are struggling with feeling unsupported. When our bones break, we feel like things are collapsing. How do you respond when you don't feel supported? Do you crumble or get stronger?

Set some goals for the month, and at the end, we will reflect on your progress. You can track your meals, exercise, appointments, and weight goals. Set some spiritual goals too.

GOALS

1. ______________________________
2. ______________________________
3. ______________________________
4. ______________________________
5. ______________________________

"Therefore encourage one another and build each other up, just as in fact you are doing."
1 Thessalonians 5:11

Monthly Affirmation:

"I am supported by God who makes me strong."

Exercise: *If you can, take the stairs instead of the elevator. Increase your daily steps goal by 10%.*

FOODS to Improve Bone Health:

- **Beans:** Cannellini, Peas
- Fat: Cottage Cheese, Ricotta
- Fruit: Tart Cherry Juice, Orange, Plantains, Papaya
- Herb: Red clover, Horsetail
- **Protein:** Turkey, Salmon, Trout, Mackerel
- **Nuts:** Almonds, Sunflower seeds, Pistachio, Chia
- Root: Sweet Potato, Carrot, Potato, Onion
- Vegetables: Broccoli, Cabbage, Okra, Collards
- Vitamins: C, D3, Glucosamine and Chondroitin, Boron

JUICE to Improve Bone Health:

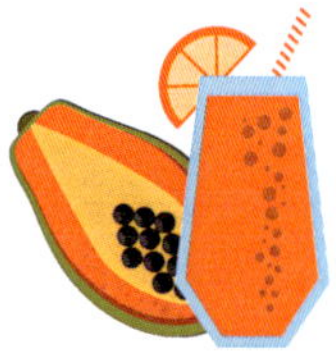

Papaya
Orange
Carrot

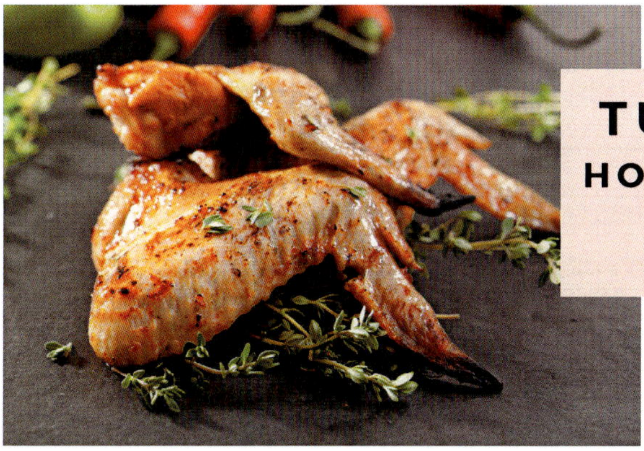

TURKEY WINGS/ HONEY-LEMON-GARLIC AND GINGER

YIELDS 2 SERVINGS

Overnight Marinade

TOTAL TIME: 45 MINS

2 - pounds of Turkey Wings
1/4 - cups of honey or agave
1 - tbsp of Minced Ginger
1 - tbsp of Minced Garlic
2 - tbsps of Tamari or soy sauce
2 - tbsps of Lemon juice
1 - tbsp of Toasted Chia seeds
1 - sprig of Rosemary
10 - ounce bag of Broccoli
1/2 - cup of water

DIRECTIONS:

- Marinate Overnight: Turkey wings in a deep baking pan with honey, lemon juice, ginger, garlic, rosemary, and Tamari sauce.
- Remove wings and save marinade.
- Place wings in baking pan. Bake for 30 minutes uncovered at 415 degrees..
- Drain fat.
- Boil marinade in sauce pan for 4 minutes.
- Pour sauce over wings, and bake at 475 degrees for 10 minutes.
- Turn wings half way until brown.
- Add 1/2 cup of water to same sauce pan
- Steam broccoli for 10 minutes covered
- Serve broccoli and Turkey wings

Medical Appointments

Date/Time Office

____

____

____

____

MEAL PLANNER * MONTH ________ YR ____

DAY 1: **MON TUES WED THU FRI SAT SUN** Cal Fat Pro Carbs

B ____________________

L ____________________

S ____________________

D ____________________

DAY 2: **MON TUES WED THU FRI SAT SUN** Cal Fat Pro Carbs

B ____________________

L ____________________

S ____________________

D ____________________

DAY 3: **MON TUES WED THU FRI SAT SUN** Cal Fat Pro Carbs

B ____________________

L ____________________

S ____________________

D ____________________

DAY 4: **MON TUES WED THU FRI SAT SUN** Cal Fat Pro Carbs

B ____________________

L ____________________

S ____________________

D ____________________

DAY 5: **MON TUES WED THU FRI SAT SUN** Cal Fat Pro Carbs

B ____________________

L ____________________

S ____________________

D ____________________

DAY 6: **MON TUES WED THU FRI SAT SUN** Cal Fat Pro Carbs

B ____________________

L ____________________

S ____________________

D ____________________

DAY 7: **MON TUES WED THU FRI SAT SUN** Cal Fat Pro Carbs

B ____________________

L ____________________

S ____________________

D ____________________

ACTIVITY PLANNER * MONTH ________ YR ____

DAY 1: MON TUES WED THU FRI SAT SUN *Time* *Calories Burned*

Exercise ______

Water ______ Steps ______

Sleep ______ Weight ______

Stress Level 0 1 2 3 4 5 6 7 8 9 10 11

DAY 2: MON TUES WED THU FRI SAT SUN *Time* *Calories Burned*

Exercise ______

Water ______ Steps ______

Sleep ______ Weight ______

Stress Level 0 1 2 3 4 5 6 7 8 9 10 11

DAY 3: MON TUES WED THU FRI SAT SUN *Time* *Calories Burned*

Exercise ______

Water ______ Steps ______

Sleep ______ Weight ______

Stress Level 0 1 2 3 4 5 6 7 8 9 10 11

DAY 4: MON TUES WED THU FRI SAT SUN *Time* *Calories Burned*

Exercise ______

Water ______ Steps ______

Sleep ______ Weight ______

Stress Level 0 1 2 3 4 5 6 7 8 9 10 11

DAY 5: MON TUES WED THU FRI SAT SUN *Time* *Calories Burned*

Exercise ______

Water ______ Steps ______

Sleep ______ Weight ______

Stress Level 0 1 2 3 4 5 6 7 8 9 10 11

DAY 6: MON TUES WED THU FRI SAT SUN *Time* *Calories Burned*

Exercise ______

Water ______ Steps ______

Sleep ______ Weight ______

Stress Level 0 1 2 3 4 5 6 7 8 9 10 11

DAY 7: MON TUES WED THU FRI SAT SUN *Time* *Calories Burned*

Exercise ______

Water ______ Steps ______

Sleep ______ Weight ______

Stress Level 0 1 2 3 4 5 6 7 8 9 10 11

MEAL PLANNER * MONTH ____ YR ____

DAY 8: **MON TUES WED THU FRI SAT SUN** Cal Fat Pro Carbs

B ____
L ____
S ____
D ____

DAY 9: **MON TUES WED THU FRI SAT SUN** Cal Fat Pro Carbs

B ____
L ____
S ____
D ____

DAY 10: **MON TUES WED THU FRI SAT SUN** Cal Fat Pro Carbs

B ____
L ____
S ____
D ____

DAY 11: **MON TUES WED THU FRI SAT SUN** Cal Fat Pro Carbs

B ____
L ____
S ____
D ____

DAY 12: **MON TUES WED THU FRI SAT SUN** Cal Fat Pro Carbs

B ____
L ____
S ____
D ____

DAY 13: **MON TUES WED THU FRI SAT SUN** Cal Fat Pro Carbs

B ____
L ____
S ____
D ____

DAY 14: **MON TUES WED THU FRI SAT SUN** Cal Fat Pro Carbs

B ____
L ____
S ____
D ____

DAY 8: **MON TUES WED THU FRI SAT SUN** *Time* *Calories Burned*

Exercise ______________________________

Water ____________ Steps ____________

Sleep ____________ Weight ____________

Stress Level 0 1 2 3 4 5 6 7 8 9 10 11

DAY 9: **MON TUES WED THU FRI SAT SUN** *Time* *Calories Burned*

Exercise ______________________________

Water ____________ Steps ____________

Sleep ____________ Weight ____________

Stress Level 0 1 2 3 4 5 6 7 8 9 10 11

DAY 10: **MON TUES WED THU FRI SAT SUN** *Time* *Calories Burned*

Exercise ______________________________

Water ____________ Steps ____________

Sleep ____________ Weight ____________

Stress Level 0 1 2 3 4 5 6 7 8 9 10 11

DAY 11: **MON TUES WED THU FRI SAT SUN** *Time* *Calories Burned*

Exercise ______________________________

Water ____________ Steps ____________

Sleep ____________ Weight ____________

Stress Level 0 1 2 3 4 5 6 7 8 9 10 11

DAY 12: **MON TUES WED THU FRI SAT SUN** *Time* *Calories Burned*

Exercise ______________________________

Water ____________ Steps ____________

Sleep ____________ Weight ____________

Stress Level 0 1 2 3 4 5 6 7 8 9 10 11

DAY 13: **MON TUES WED THU FRI SAT SUN** *Time* *Calories Burned*

Exercise ______________________________

Water ____________ Steps ____________

Sleep ____________ Weight ____________

Stress Level 0 1 2 3 4 5 6 7 8 9 10 11

DAY 14: **MON TUES WED THU FRI SAT SUN** *Time* *Calories Burned*

Exercise ______________________________

Water ____________ Steps ____________

Sleep ____________ Weight ____________

Stress Level 0 1 2 3 4 5 6 7 8 9 10 11

MEAL PLANNER * MONTH ________ YR ____

DAY 15: **MON TUES WED THU FRI SAT SUN** Cal Fat Pro Carbs

B ____

L ____

S ____

D ____

DAY 16: **MON TUES WED THU FRI SAT SUN** Cal Fat Pro Carbs

B ____

L ____

S ____

D ____

DAY 17: **MON TUES WED THU FRI SAT SUN** Cal Fat Pro Carbs

B ____

L ____

S ____

D ____

DAY 18: **MON TUES WED THU FRI SAT SUN** Cal Fat Pro Carbs

B ____

L ____

S ____

D ____

DAY 19: **MON TUES WED THU FRI SAT SUN** Cal Fat Pro Carbs

B ____

L ____

S ____

D ____

DAY 20: **MON TUES WED THU FRI SAT SUN** Cal Fat Pro Carbs

B ____

L ____

S ____

D ____

DAY 21: **MON TUES WED THU FRI SAT SUN** Cal Fat Pro Carbs

B ____

L ____

S ____

D ____

DAY 15: **MON TUES WED THU FRI SAT SUN** *Time* *Calories Burned*

Exercise ____________________

Water __________ Steps __________

Sleep __________ Weight __________

Stress Level 0 1 2 3 4 5 6 7 8 9 10 11

DAY 16: **MON TUES WED THU FRI SAT SUN** *Time* *Calories Burned*

Exercise ____________________

Water __________ Steps __________

Sleep __________ Weight __________

Stress Level 0 1 2 3 4 5 6 7 8 9 10 11

DAY 17: **MON TUES WED THU FRI SAT SUN** *Time* *Calories Burned*

Exercise ____________________

Water __________ Steps __________

Sleep __________ Weight __________

Stress Level 0 1 2 3 4 5 6 7 8 9 10 11

DAY 18: **MON TUES WED THU FRI SAT SUN** *Time* *Calories Burned*

Exercise ____________________

Water __________ Steps __________

Sleep __________ Weight __________

Stress Level 0 1 2 3 4 5 6 7 8 9 10 11

DAY 19: **MON TUES WED THU FRI SAT SUN** *Time* *Calories Burned*

Exercise ____________________

Water __________ Steps __________

Sleep __________ Weight __________

Stress Level 0 1 2 3 4 5 6 7 8 9 10 11

DAY 20: **MON TUES WED THU FRI SAT SUN** *Time* *Calories Burned*

Exercise ____________________

Water __________ Steps __________

Sleep __________ Weight __________

Stress Level 0 1 2 3 4 5 6 7 8 9 10 11

DAY 21: **MON TUES WED THU FRI SAT SUN** *Time* *Calories Burned*

Exercise ____________________

Water __________ Steps __________

Sleep __________ Weight __________

Stress Level 0 1 2 3 4 5 6 7 8 9 10 11

DAY 22: MON TUES WED THU FRI SAT SUN Cal Fat Pro Carbs

B ____
L ____
S ____
D ____

DAY 23: MON TUES WED THU FRI SAT SUN Cal Fat Pro Carbs

B ____
L ____
S ____
D ____

DAY 24: MON TUES WED THU FRI SAT SUN Cal Fat Pro Carbs

B ____
L ____
S ____
D ____

DAY 25: MON TUES WED THU FRI SAT SUN Cal Fat Pro Carbs

B ____
L ____
S ____
D ____

DAY 26: MON TUES WED THU FRI SAT SUN Cal Fat Pro Carbs

B ____
L ____
S ____
D ____

DAY 27: MON TUES WED THU FRI SAT SUN Cal Fat Pro Carbs

B ____
L ____
S ____
D ____

DAY 28: MON TUES WED THU FRI SAT SUN Cal Fat Pro Carbs

B ____
L ____
S ____
D ____

DAY 22: **MON TUES WED THU FRI SAT SUN** *Time* *Calories Burned*

Exercise ______

Water ______ Steps ______

Sleep ______ Weight ______

Stress Level 0 1 2 3 4 5 6 7 8 9 10 11

DAY 23: **MON TUES WED THU FRI SAT SUN** *Time* *Calories Burned*

Exercise ______

Water ______ Steps ______

Sleep ______ Weight ______

Stress Level 0 1 2 3 4 5 6 7 8 9 10 11

DAY 24: **MON TUES WED THU FRI SAT SUN** *Time* *Calories Burned*

Exercise ______

Water ______ Steps ______

Sleep ______ Weight ______

Stress Level 0 1 2 3 4 5 6 7 8 9 10 11

DAY 25: **MON TUES WED THU FRI SAT SUN** *Time* *Calories Burned*

Exercise ______

Water ______ Steps ______

Sleep ______ Weight ______

Stress Level 0 1 2 3 4 5 6 7 8 9 10 11

DAY 26: **MON TUES WED THU FRI SAT SUN** *Time* *Calories Burned*

Exercise ______

Water ______ Steps ______

Sleep ______ Weight ______

Stress Level 0 1 2 3 4 5 6 7 8 9 10 11

DAY 27: **MON TUES WED THU FRI SAT SUN** *Time* *Calories Burned*

Exercise ______

Water ______ Steps ______

Sleep ______ Weight ______

Stress Level 0 1 2 3 4 5 6 7 8 9 10 11

DAY 28: **MON TUES WED THU FRI SAT SUN** *Time* *Calories Burned*

Exercise ______

Water ______ Steps ______

Sleep ______ Weight ______

Stress Level 0 1 2 3 4 5 6 7 8 9 10 11

MEAL PLANNER * MONTH ______ YR ______

DAY 29: **MON TUES WED THU FRI SAT SUN** Cal Fat Pro Carbs

B ____________________

L ____________________

S ____________________

D ____________________

DAY 30: **MON TUES WED THU FRI SAT SUN** Cal Fat Pro Carbs

B ____________________

L ____________________

S ____________________

D ____________________

DAY 31: **MON TUES WED THU FRI SAT SUN** Cal Fat Pro Carbs

B ____________________

L ____________________

S ____________________

D ____________________

GOALS

	Achieved Y	N
1. ____________________	☐	☐
2. ____________________	☐	☐
3. ____________________	☐	☐
4. ____________________	☐	☐
5. ____________________	☐	☐

End of Month Results

Weight | *Blood Pressure* | *Resting Heart Rate*

DAY 29: **MON TUES WED THU FRI SAT SUN** *Time* *Calories Burned*

Exercise ____

Water ____________________ Steps ____________________

Sleep ____________________ Weight ____________________

Stress Level 0 1 2 3 4 5 6 7 8 9 10 11

DAY 30: **MON TUES WED THU FRI SAT SUN** *Time* *Calories Burned*

Exercise ____

Water ____________________ Steps ____________________

Sleep ____________________ Weight ____________________

Stress Level 0 1 2 3 4 5 6 7 8 9 10 11

DAY 31: **MON TUES WED THU FRI SAT SUN** *Time* *Calories Burned*

Exercise ____

Water ____________________ Steps ____________________

Sleep ____________________ Weight ____________________

Stress Level 0 1 2 3 4 5 6 7 8 9 10 11

STRESSORS

	Resolved Y	Resolved N
1. ______________________	☐	☐
2. ______________________	☐	☐
3. ______________________	☐	☐
4. ______________________	☐	☐
5. ______________________	☐	☐

of Successful Days

Count all the days this month you achieved your own health goals.

Exercise ◯ Water ◯ Steps ◯ Sleep ◯ Weight ◯

ACTIVITY PLANNER * MONTH ________ YR ____

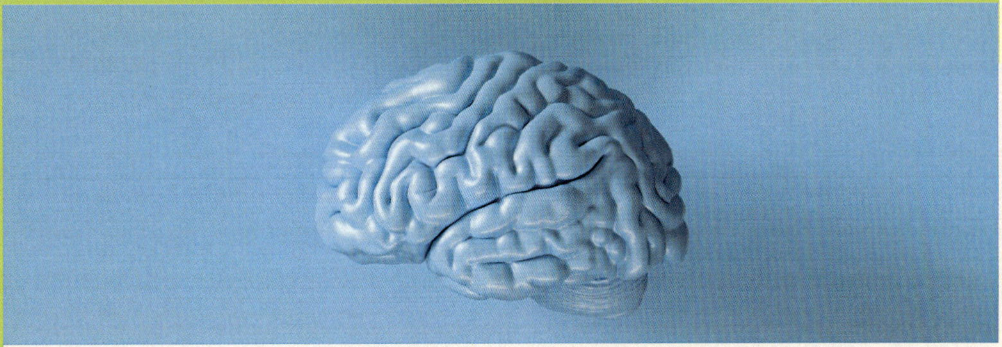

6. BRAIN

Alzheimer's, Dementia, Parkinson's
Mental Illness, Depression, Anxiety

Those who suffer from mental illness are under attack spiritually. There is always a spiritual component to all physical and mental illnesses. For example, Alzheimer's is the fear of the future/death. Dementia is denial of the past. Depression is anger and sadness about the past. Anxiety is fear of the future, most of which is self-induced, as an escape from the present.

Set some goals for the month, and at the end, we will reflect on your progress. You can track your meals, exercise, appointments, and weight goals. Set some spiritual goals too.

GOALS

1. ______________________________
2. ______________________________
3. ______________________________
4. ______________________________
5. ______________________________

"Fear thou not; for I am with thee: be not dismayed; for I am thy God: I will strengthen thee; yea, I will help thee; yea, I will uphold thee with the right hand of my righteousness."
Isaiah 41:10

Monthly Affirmation:

"I am embracing the present moment."

Exercise: *When you drink your tea, or eat your food, pay more attention to every sip or bite over all else.*

FOODS to Improve Brain Health:

- **Beans:** Navy, Kidney, Black, Lentils
- Fat: Whole Eggs, Almond Butter, Coconut Oil
- Fruit: Avocado, Cherry Tomato, Blueberries
- Herb: Green Tea, Curry, Turmeric, Chamomile
- **Protein:** Salmon, Non-canned Tuna, Chicken, Tofu
- **Nuts:** Walnuts, Pumpkin Seeds, Sunflower Seeds
- Root: Rutabaga, Purple Sweet Potato
- Vegetables: Red Cabbage, Kale, Spinach, Broccoli, Collard Greens
- Vitamins: B2, B6, B9, B12, D, E, CoQ10, Magnesium
- Grains: Quinoa, Brown Rice, Black Rice

JUICE to Improve Brain Health:

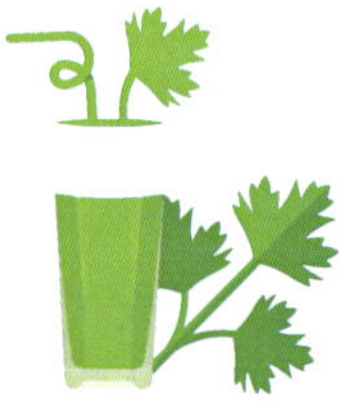

Apple
Cranberry
Parsley

Contact Vandene:
for Local South Florida Delivery
ordersmavis@gmail.com

M.A.V.I.S
Health Drinks

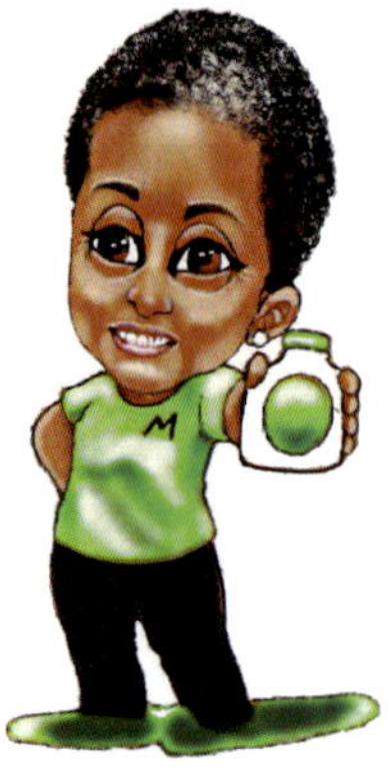

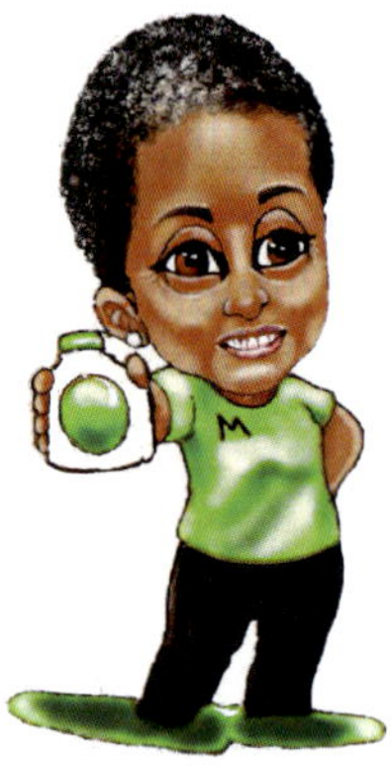

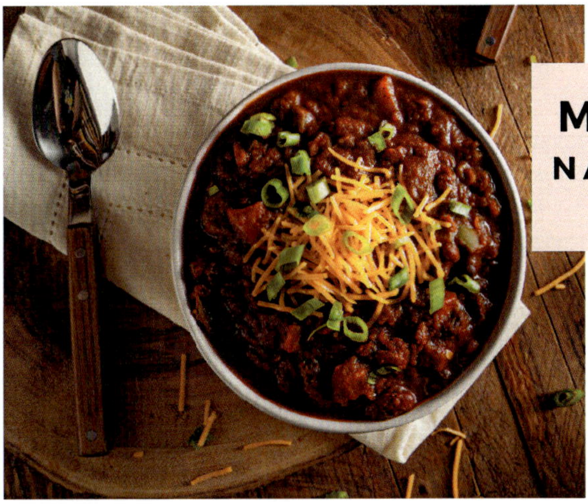

MEATLESS CHILI

NAVY, KIDNEY, LENTIL

YIELDS 4 SERVINGS

TOTAL TIME: 45 MINS

2 - tbsp olive oil
1 - Red bell pepper - diced
1 - small diced Onion
2 - cloves Garlic - minced
2 - tsp of Chili powder
1 - tsp of Ground Cayenne pepper
1 - tsp of Ground Cumin
1 - tsp of Kosher sea salt
1 - tsp of ground black pepper
2/3 - cup Tomato sauce
1 - can of diced Tomatoes
1 - cup of water
1 - can of Navy beans
1 - can of Kidney beans
1 - cup of Dried Lentils
1 - Scallion, chopped

DIRECTIONS:

- Heat Large stock pot to Medium-High heat
- Add oil, bell pepper, onions, and garlic
- Cook for 5 minutes
- Add chili powder, cayenne, cumin, salt, pepper. Stir well. Cook for 3 minutes.
- Add tomato sauce and diced tomatoes, and stir continuously for 1 minute
- Add water and bring to a boil
- Add Navy beans, kidney beans, and lentils
- Reduce heat to a simmer for 30 minutes
- For softer lentils, add 10 minutes
- Serve chili and top with chopped scallion and shredded cheese (optional)

Medical Appointments

Date/Time	Office

MEAL PLANNER * MONTH ________ YR ____

DAY 1: MON TUES WED THU FRI SAT SUN Cal Fat Pro Carbs

B ____________________

L ____________________

S ____________________

D ____________________

DAY 2: MON TUES WED THU FRI SAT SUN Cal Fat Pro Carbs

B ____________________

L ____________________

S ____________________

D ____________________

DAY 3: MON TUES WED THU FRI SAT SUN Cal Fat Pro Carbs

B ____________________

L ____________________

S ____________________

D ____________________

DAY 4: MON TUES WED THU FRI SAT SUN Cal Fat Pro Carbs

B ____________________

L ____________________

S ____________________

D ____________________

DAY 5: MON TUES WED THU FRI SAT SUN Cal Fat Pro Carbs

B ____________________

L ____________________

S ____________________

D ____________________

DAY 6: MON TUES WED THU FRI SAT SUN Cal Fat Pro Carbs

B ____________________

L ____________________

S ____________________

D ____________________

DAY 7: MON TUES WED THU FRI SAT SUN Cal Fat Pro Carbs

B ____________________

L ____________________

S ____________________

D ____________________

ACTIVITY PLANNER * MONTH ________ YR ____

DAY 1: MON TUES WED THU FRI SAT SUN *Time* *Calories Burned*

Exercise ____________________

Water ____________ Steps ____________

Sleep ____________ Weight ____________

Stress Level 0 1 2 3 4 5 6 7 8 9 10 11

DAY 2: MON TUES WED THU FRI SAT SUN *Time* *Calories Burned*

Exercise ____________________

Water ____________ Steps ____________

Sleep ____________ Weight ____________

Stress Level 0 1 2 3 4 5 6 7 8 9 10 11

DAY 3: MON TUES WED THU FRI SAT SUN *Time* *Calories Burned*

Exercise ____________________

Water ____________ Steps ____________

Sleep ____________ Weight ____________

Stress Level 0 1 2 3 4 5 6 7 8 9 10 11

DAY 4: MON TUES WED THU FRI SAT SUN *Time* *Calories Burned*

Exercise ____________________

Water ____________ Steps ____________

Sleep ____________ Weight ____________

Stress Level 0 1 2 3 4 5 6 7 8 9 10 11

DAY 5: MON TUES WED THU FRI SAT SUN *Time* *Calories Burned*

Exercise ____________________

Water ____________ Steps ____________

Sleep ____________ Weight ____________

Stress Level 0 1 2 3 4 5 6 7 8 9 10 11

DAY 6: MON TUES WED THU FRI SAT SUN *Time* *Calories Burned*

Exercise ____________________

Water ____________ Steps ____________

Sleep ____________ Weight ____________

Stress Level 0 1 2 3 4 5 6 7 8 9 10 11

DAY 7: MON TUES WED THU FRI SAT SUN *Time* *Calories Burned*

Exercise ____________________

Water ____________ Steps ____________

Sleep ____________ Weight ____________

Stress Level 0 1 2 3 4 5 6 7 8 9 10 11

DAY 8: **MON TUES WED THU FRI SAT SUN** Cal Fat Pro Carbs

B ____________________

L ____________________

S ____________________

D ____________________

DAY 9: **MON TUES WED THU FRI SAT SUN** Cal Fat Pro Carbs

B ____________________

L ____________________

S ____________________

D ____________________

DAY 10: **MON TUES WED THU FRI SAT SUN** Cal Fat Pro Carbs

B ____________________

L ____________________

S ____________________

D ____________________

DAY 11: **MON TUES WED THU FRI SAT SUN** Cal Fat Pro Carbs

B ____________________

L ____________________

S ____________________

D ____________________

DAY 12: **MON TUES WED THU FRI SAT SUN** Cal Fat Pro Carbs

B ____________________

L ____________________

S ____________________

D ____________________

DAY 13: **MON TUES WED THU FRI SAT SUN** Cal Fat Pro Carbs

B ____________________

L ____________________

S ____________________

D ____________________

DAY 14: **MON TUES WED THU FRI SAT SUN** Cal Fat Pro Carbs

B ____________________

L ____________________

S ____________________

D ____________________

DAY 8: **MON TUES WED THU FRI SAT SUN** *Time* *Calories Burned*

Exercise ______

Water ______ Steps ______

Sleep ______ Weight ______

Stress Level 0 1 2 3 4 5 6 7 8 9 10 11

DAY 9: **MON TUES WED THU FRI SAT SUN** *Time* *Calories Burned*

Exercise ______

Water ______ Steps ______

Sleep ______ Weight ______

Stress Level 0 1 2 3 4 5 6 7 8 9 10 11

DAY 10: **MON TUES WED THU FRI SAT SUN** *Time* *Calories Burned*

Exercise ______

Water ______ Steps ______

Sleep ______ Weight ______

Stress Level 0 1 2 3 4 5 6 7 8 9 10 11

DAY 11: **MON TUES WED THU FRI SAT SUN** *Time* *Calories Burned*

Exercise ______

Water ______ Steps ______

Sleep ______ Weight ______

Stress Level 0 1 2 3 4 5 6 7 8 9 10 11

DAY 12: **MON TUES WED THU FRI SAT SUN** *Time* *Calories Burned*

Exercise ______

Water ______ Steps ______

Sleep ______ Weight ______

Stress Level 0 1 2 3 4 5 6 7 8 9 10 11

DAY 13: **MON TUES WED THU FRI SAT SUN** *Time* *Calories Burned*

Exercise ______

Water ______ Steps ______

Sleep ______ Weight ______

Stress Level 0 1 2 3 4 5 6 7 8 9 10 11

DAY 14: **MON TUES WED THU FRI SAT SUN** *Time* *Calories Burned*

Exercise ______

Water ______ Steps ______

Sleep ______ Weight ______

Stress Level 0 1 2 3 4 5 6 7 8 9 10 11

DAY 15: MON TUES WED THU FRI SAT SUN Cal Fat Pro Carbs

B ______

L ______

S ______

D ______

DAY 16: MON TUES WED THU FRI SAT SUN Cal Fat Pro Carbs

B ______

L ______

S ______

D ______

DAY 17: MON TUES WED THU FRI SAT SUN Cal Fat Pro Carbs

B ______

L ______

S ______

D ______

DAY 18: MON TUES WED THU FRI SAT SUN Cal Fat Pro Carbs

B ______

L ______

S ______

D ______

DAY 19: MON TUES WED THU FRI SAT SUN Cal Fat Pro Carbs

B ______

L ______

S ______

D ______

DAY 20: MON TUES WED THU FRI SAT SUN Cal Fat Pro Carbs

B ______

L ______

S ______

D ______

DAY 21: MON TUES WED THU FRI SAT SUN Cal Fat Pro Carbs

B ______

L ______

S ______

D ______

DAY 15: **MON TUES WED THU FRI SAT SUN** *Time* *Calories Burned*

Exercise ________________________________

Water ________________ Steps ________________

Sleep ________________ Weight ________________

Stress Level 0 1 2 3 4 5 6 7 8 9 10 11

DAY 16: **MON TUES WED THU FRI SAT SUN** *Time* *Calories Burned*

Exercise ________________________________

Water ________________ Steps ________________

Sleep ________________ Weight ________________

Stress Level 0 1 2 3 4 5 6 7 8 9 10 11

DAY 17: **MON TUES WED THU FRI SAT SUN** *Time* *Calories Burned*

Exercise ________________________________

Water ________________ Steps ________________

Sleep ________________ Weight ________________

Stress Level 0 1 2 3 4 5 6 7 8 9 10 11

DAY 18: **MON TUES WED THU FRI SAT SUN** *Time* *Calories Burned*

Exercise ________________________________

Water ________________ Steps ________________

Sleep ________________ Weight ________________

Stress Level 0 1 2 3 4 5 6 7 8 9 10 11

DAY 19: **MON TUES WED THU FRI SAT SUN** *Time* *Calories Burned*

Exercise ________________________________

Water ________________ Steps ________________

Sleep ________________ Weight ________________

Stress Level 0 1 2 3 4 5 6 7 8 9 10 11

DAY 20: **MON TUES WED THU FRI SAT SUN** *Time* *Calories Burned*

Exercise ________________________________

Water ________________ Steps ________________

Sleep ________________ Weight ________________

Stress Level 0 1 2 3 4 5 6 7 8 9 10 11

DAY 21: **MON TUES WED THU FRI SAT SUN** *Time* *Calories Burned*

Exercise ________________________________

Water ________________ Steps ________________

Sleep ________________ Weight ________________

Stress Level 0 1 2 3 4 5 6 7 8 9 10 11

MEAL PLANNER * MONTH ________ YR ____

DAY 22: MON TUES WED THU FRI SAT SUN Cal Fat Pro Carbs

B ____
L ____
S ____
D ____

DAY 23: MON TUES WED THU FRI SAT SUN Cal Fat Pro Carbs

B ____
L ____
S ____
D ____

DAY 24: MON TUES WED THU FRI SAT SUN Cal Fat Pro Carbs

B ____
L ____
S ____
D ____

DAY 25: MON TUES WED THU FRI SAT SUN Cal Fat Pro Carbs

B ____
L ____
S ____
D ____

DAY 26: MON TUES WED THU FRI SAT SUN Cal Fat Pro Carbs

B ____
L ____
S ____
D ____

DAY 27: MON TUES WED THU FRI SAT SUN Cal Fat Pro Carbs

B ____
L ____
S ____
D ____

DAY 28: MON TUES WED THU FRI SAT SUN Cal Fat Pro Carbs

B ____
L ____
S ____
D ____

DAY 22: **MON TUES WED THU FRI SAT SUN** *Time* *Calories Burned*

Exercise ____________________

Water ____________ Steps ____________

Sleep ____________ Weight ____________

Stress Level 0 1 2 3 4 5 6 7 8 9 10 11

DAY 23: **MON TUES WED THU FRI SAT SUN** *Time* *Calories Burned*

Exercise ____________________

Water ____________ Steps ____________

Sleep ____________ Weight ____________

Stress Level 0 1 2 3 4 5 6 7 8 9 10 11

DAY 24: **MON TUES WED THU FRI SAT SUN** *Time* *Calories Burned*

Exercise ____________________

Water ____________ Steps ____________

Sleep ____________ Weight ____________

Stress Level 0 1 2 3 4 5 6 7 8 9 10 11

DAY 25: **MON TUES WED THU FRI SAT SUN** *Time* *Calories Burned*

Exercise ____________________

Water ____________ Steps ____________

Sleep ____________ Weight ____________

Stress Level 0 1 2 3 4 5 6 7 8 9 10 11

DAY 26: **MON TUES WED THU FRI SAT SUN** *Time* *Calories Burned*

Exercise ____________________

Water ____________ Steps ____________

Sleep ____________ Weight ____________

Stress Level 0 1 2 3 4 5 6 7 8 9 10 11

DAY 27: **MON TUES WED THU FRI SAT SUN** *Time* *Calories Burned*

Exercise ____________________

Water ____________ Steps ____________

Sleep ____________ Weight ____________

Stress Level 0 1 2 3 4 5 6 7 8 9 10 11

DAY 28: **MON TUES WED THU FRI SAT SUN** *Time* *Calories Burned*

Exercise ____________________

Water ____________ Steps ____________

Sleep ____________ Weight ____________

Stress Level 0 1 2 3 4 5 6 7 8 9 10 11

MEAL PLANNER * MONTH ________ YR ______

DAY 29: **MON TUES WED THU FRI SAT SUN** Cal Fat Pro Carbs

B ____________________

L ____________________

S ____________________

D ____________________

DAY 30: **MON TUES WED THU FRI SAT SUN** Cal Fat Pro Carbs

B ____________________

L ____________________

S ____________________

D ____________________

DAY 31: **MON TUES WED THU FRI SAT SUN** Cal Fat Pro Carbs

B ____________________

L ____________________

S ____________________

D ____________________

GOALS

Achieved Y N

1. ____________________ ☐ ☐
2. ____________________ ☐ ☐
3. ____________________ ☐ ☐
4. ____________________ ☐ ☐
5. ____________________ ☐ ☐

End of Month Results

Weight

Blood Pressure

Resting Heart Rate

DAY 29: **MON TUES WED THU FRI SAT SUN** *Time* *Calories Burned*

Exercise ______________________________

Water ______________ Steps ______________

Sleep ______________ Weight ______________

Stress Level 0 1 2 3 4 5 6 7 8 9 10 11

DAY 30: **MON TUES WED THU FRI SAT SUN** *Time* *Calories Burned*

Exercise ______________________________

Water ______________ Steps ______________

Sleep ______________ Weight ______________

Stress Level 0 1 2 3 4 5 6 7 8 9 10 11

DAY 31: **MON TUES WED THU FRI SAT SUN** *Time* *Calories Burned*

Exercise ______________________________

Water ______________ Steps ______________

Sleep ______________ Weight ______________

Stress Level 0 1 2 3 4 5 6 7 8 9 10 11

STRESSORS

	Resolved Y	Resolved N
1. ______________	☐	☐
2. ______________	☐	☐
3. ______________	☐	☐
4. ______________	☐	☐
5. ______________	☐	☐

of Successful Days

Count all the days this month you achieved your own health goals.

Exercise ◯ Water ◯ Steps ◯ Sleep ◯ Weight ◯

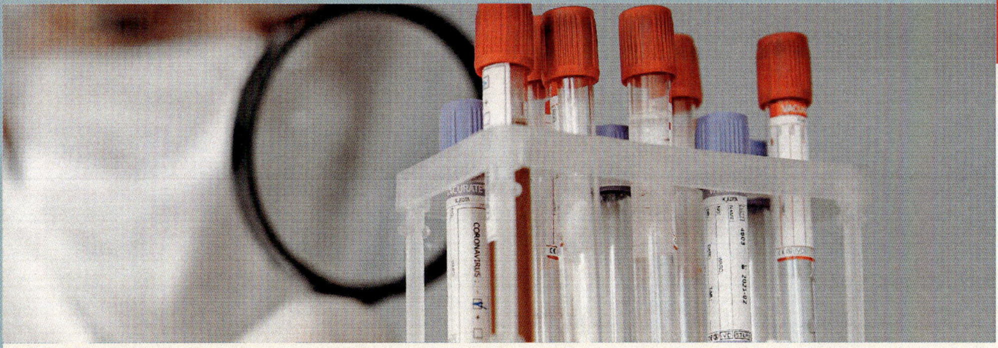

7. BLOOD

Red Blood Cells, Plasma, Platelets

Think of the blood as a highway, that transports oxygen-poor blood into the heart, and oxygenates it. Then, it pumps the oxygen-rich blood out of the heart, carrying nutrients and toxins away from the heart to the rest of the body. It passes through the lymph system to be purified, and sends good blood back to the heart. The other organs receive this good blood (aka joy). Problems with the blood are related to an inability to find joy. If the blood is not purified, the organs will get "bad blood". That "bad blood" will return to the heart. Now, you understand why people stay broken-hearted. It's because of "bad blood". Not letting go of toxic thinking.

Set some goals for the month, and at the end, we will reflect on your progress. You can track your meals, exercise, appointments, and weight goals. Set some spiritual goals too.

GOALS

1. ______________________________
2. ______________________________
3. ______________________________
4. ______________________________
5. ______________________________

"For there are three that testify: the Spirit and the water and the blood; and these three agree."
1 John 4:7,8

Monthly Affirmation:

"I am finding joy in everything I do."

Exercise: *Find a place that gives you joy. Make it a point to go to this place. Intentionally* ***find*** *your joy.*

FOODS to Improve Blood Health:

- **Beans:** Lima, Pinto, White, Edamame
- **Fat:** Yogurt, Safflower Oil
- **Fruit:** Blueberries, Grapes, Apples, Prunes
- **Herb:** Garlic, Turmeric, Green Tea, Spirulina
- **Protein:** Cod, Saith, Haddock
- **Nuts:** Almonds, Cashews
- **Root:** Yam, Beets, Raw Carrot
- **Vegetables:** Cauliflower, Artichoke, Eggplant, Brussels
- **Vitamins:** Potassium, Calcium, Magnesium, Folate, Iron
- **Grains:** Oatmeal, Oat Bran, Pumpernickel

JUICE to Improve Blood Health:

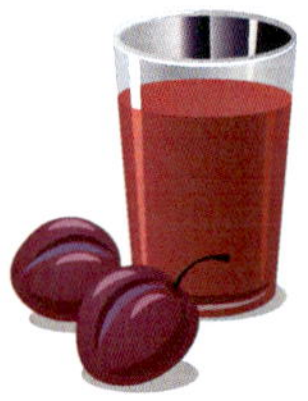

Apple
Prune
Berry

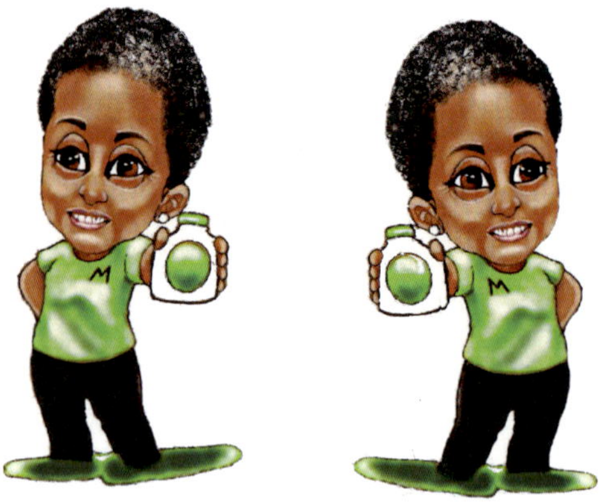

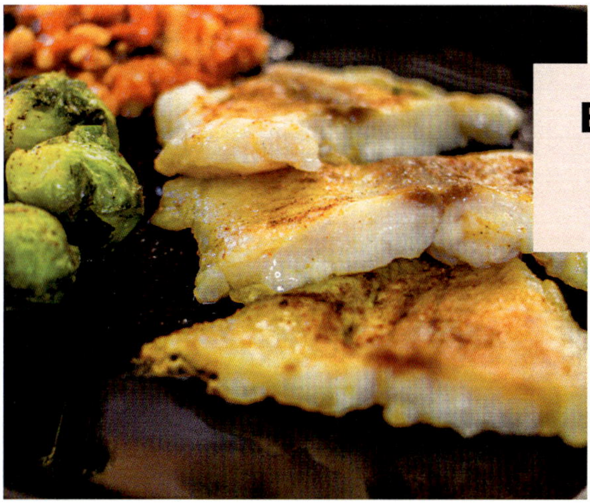

BAKED COD W/ BRUSSEL SPROUTS

YIELDS 4 SERVINGS

TOTAL TIME: 35 MINS

4 - Cod fillets
1 - pound of Brussels sprouts, halved
2 - cloves of Garlic, mined
1 - tsp of Ground Cumin
1 - tsp of Onion powder
1 - tsp of sea salt (use in 2 parts)
1 - dash of crushed pepper
4 - tbsp of Olive Oil (use in 2 parts)
1 - Lemon (juiced) w/zest
1 - Pumpernickel Loaf

DIRECTIONS:

- Preheat over to 400 degrees F
- In a bowl, mix crushed pepper, cumin, garlic, olive oil, lemon juice, sea salt
- In a baking pan, line with baking paper and lightly grease with olive oil
- Put cod fillets in the center
- Spread mixture over cods
- Place Brussel sprouts around the cod
- Drizzle with sea salt, lemon zest, and oil
- Bake for 20 minutes
- Toast slices of Pumpernickel loaf
- Serve with cod, Brussel sprouts and toast

Medical Appointments

Date/Time Office

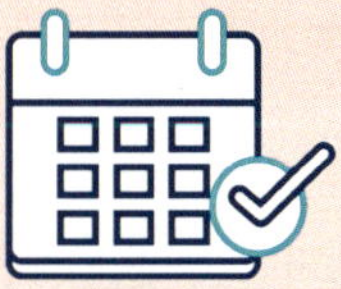

MEAL PLANNER * MONTH ______ YR ____

DAY 1: **MON TUES WED THU FRI SAT SUN** Cal Fat Pro Carbs

B ____
L ____
S ____
D ____

DAY 2: **MON TUES WED THU FRI SAT SUN** Cal Fat Pro Carbs

B ____
L ____
S ____
D ____

DAY 3: **MON TUES WED THU FRI SAT SUN** Cal Fat Pro Carbs

B ____
L ____
S ____
D ____

DAY 4: **MON TUES WED THU FRI SAT SUN** Cal Fat Pro Carbs

B ____
L ____
S ____
D ____

DAY 5: **MON TUES WED THU FRI SAT SUN** Cal Fat Pro Carbs

B ____
L ____
S ____
D ____

DAY 6: **MON TUES WED THU FRI SAT SUN** Cal Fat Pro Carbs

B ____
L ____
S ____
D ____

DAY 7: **MON TUES WED THU FRI SAT SUN** Cal Fat Pro Carbs

B ____
L ____
S ____
D ____

ACTIVITY PLANNER * MONTH ________ YR ____

DAY 1: **MON TUES WED THU FRI SAT SUN** *Time* *Calories Burned*

Exercise ____________________

Water ____________ Steps ____________

Sleep ____________ Weight ____________

Stress Level 0 1 2 3 4 5 6 7 8 9 10 11

DAY 2: **MON TUES WED THU FRI SAT SUN** *Time* *Calories Burned*

Exercise ____________________

Water ____________ Steps ____________

Sleep ____________ Weight ____________

Stress Level 0 1 2 3 4 5 6 7 8 9 10 11

DAY 3: **MON TUES WED THU FRI SAT SUN** *Time* *Calories Burned*

Exercise ____________________

Water ____________ Steps ____________

Sleep ____________ Weight ____________

Stress Level 0 1 2 3 4 5 6 7 8 9 10 11

DAY 4: **MON TUES WED THU FRI SAT SUN** *Time* *Calories Burned*

Exercise ____________________

Water ____________ Steps ____________

Sleep ____________ Weight ____________

Stress Level 0 1 2 3 4 5 6 7 8 9 10 11

DAY 5: **MON TUES WED THU FRI SAT SUN** *Time* *Calories Burned*

Exercise ____________________

Water ____________ Steps ____________

Sleep ____________ Weight ____________

Stress Level 0 1 2 3 4 5 6 7 8 9 10 11

DAY 6: **MON TUES WED THU FRI SAT SUN** *Time* *Calories Burned*

Exercise ____________________

Water ____________ Steps ____________

Sleep ____________ Weight ____________

Stress Level 0 1 2 3 4 5 6 7 8 9 10 11

DAY 7: **MON TUES WED THU FRI SAT SUN** *Time* *Calories Burned*

Exercise ____________________

Water ____________ Steps ____________

Sleep ____________ Weight ____________

Stress Level 0 1 2 3 4 5 6 7 8 9 10 11

MEAL PLANNER * MONTH ___ YR ___

DAY 8: **MON TUES WED THU FRI SAT SUN** Cal Fat Pro Carbs

B ____

L ____

S ____

D ____

DAY 9: **MON TUES WED THU FRI SAT SUN** Cal Fat Pro Carbs

B ____

L ____

S ____

D ____

DAY 10: **MON TUES WED THU FRI SAT SUN** Cal Fat Pro Carbs

B ____

L ____

S ____

D ____

DAY 11: **MON TUES WED THU FRI SAT SUN** Cal Fat Pro Carbs

B ____

L ____

S ____

D ____

DAY 12: **MON TUES WED THU FRI SAT SUN** Cal Fat Pro Carbs

B ____

L ____

S ____

D ____

DAY 13: **MON TUES WED THU FRI SAT SUN** Cal Fat Pro Carbs

B ____

L ____

S ____

D ____

DAY 14: **MON TUES WED THU FRI SAT SUN** Cal Fat Pro Carbs

B ____

L ____

S ____

D ____

DAY 8: **MON TUES WED THU FRI SAT SUN** *Time* *Calories Burned*

Exercise ______________________________

Water ______________ Steps ______________

Sleep ______________ Weight ______________

Stress Level 0 1 2 3 4 5 6 7 8 9 10 11

DAY 9: **MON TUES WED THU FRI SAT SUN** *Time* *Calories Burned*

Exercise ______________________________

Water ______________ Steps ______________

Sleep ______________ Weight ______________

Stress Level 0 1 2 3 4 5 6 7 8 9 10 11

DAY 10: **MON TUES WED THU FRI SAT SUN** *Time* *Calories Burned*

Exercise ______________________________

Water ______________ Steps ______________

Sleep ______________ Weight ______________

Stress Level 0 1 2 3 4 5 6 7 8 9 10 11

DAY 11: **MON TUES WED THU FRI SAT SUN** *Time* *Calories Burned*

Exercise ______________________________

Water ______________ Steps ______________

Sleep ______________ Weight ______________

Stress Level 0 1 2 3 4 5 6 7 8 9 10 11

DAY 12: **MON TUES WED THU FRI SAT SUN** *Time* *Calories Burned*

Exercise ______________________________

Water ______________ Steps ______________

Sleep ______________ Weight ______________

Stress Level 0 1 2 3 4 5 6 7 8 9 10 11

DAY 13: **MON TUES WED THU FRI SAT SUN** *Time* *Calories Burned*

Exercise ______________________________

Water ______________ Steps ______________

Sleep ______________ Weight ______________

Stress Level 0 1 2 3 4 5 6 7 8 9 10 11

DAY 14: **MON TUES WED THU FRI SAT SUN** *Time* *Calories Burned*

Exercise ______________________________

Water ______________ Steps ______________

Sleep ______________ Weight ______________

Stress Level 0 1 2 3 4 5 6 7 8 9 10 11

MEAL PLANNER * MONTH ________ YR ______

DAY 15: **MON TUES WED THU FRI SAT SUN** Cal Fat Pro Carbs

B ______

L ______

S ______

D ______

DAY 16: **MON TUES WED THU FRI SAT SUN** Cal Fat Pro Carbs

B ______

L ______

S ______

D ______

DAY 17: **MON TUES WED THU FRI SAT SUN** Cal Fat Pro Carbs

B ______

L ______

S ______

D ______

DAY 18: **MON TUES WED THU FRI SAT SUN** Cal Fat Pro Carbs

B ______

L ______

S ______

D ______

DAY 19: **MON TUES WED THU FRI SAT SUN** Cal Fat Pro Carbs

B ______

L ______

S ______

D ______

DAY 20: **MON TUES WED THU FRI SAT SUN** Cal Fat Pro Carbs

B ______

L ______

S ______

D ______

DAY 21: **MON TUES WED THU FRI SAT SUN** Cal Fat Pro Carbs

B ______

L ______

S ______

D ______

DAY 15: **MON TUES WED THU FRI SAT SUN** *Time* *Calories Burned*

Exercise ________________________________

Water ______________ Steps ______________

Sleep ______________ Weight ______________

Stress Level 0 1 2 3 4 5 6 7 8 9 10 11

DAY 16: **MON TUES WED THU FRI SAT SUN** *Time* *Calories Burned*

Exercise ________________________________

Water ______________ Steps ______________

Sleep ______________ Weight ______________

Stress Level 0 1 2 3 4 5 6 7 8 9 10 11

DAY 17: **MON TUES WED THU FRI SAT SUN** *Time* *Calories Burned*

Exercise ________________________________

Water ______________ Steps ______________

Sleep ______________ Weight ______________

Stress Level 0 1 2 3 4 5 6 7 8 9 10 11

DAY 18: **MON TUES WED THU FRI SAT SUN** *Time* *Calories Burned*

Exercise ________________________________

Water ______________ Steps ______________

Sleep ______________ Weight ______________

Stress Level 0 1 2 3 4 5 6 7 8 9 10 11

DAY 19: **MON TUES WED THU FRI SAT SUN** *Time* *Calories Burned*

Exercise ________________________________

Water ______________ Steps ______________

Sleep ______________ Weight ______________

Stress Level 0 1 2 3 4 5 6 7 8 9 10 11

DAY 20: **MON TUES WED THU FRI SAT SUN** *Time* *Calories Burned*

Exercise ________________________________

Water ______________ Steps ______________

Sleep ______________ Weight ______________

Stress Level 0 1 2 3 4 5 6 7 8 9 10 11

DAY 21: **MON TUES WED THU FRI SAT SUN** *Time* *Calories Burned*

Exercise ________________________________

Water ______________ Steps ______________

Sleep ______________ Weight ______________

Stress Level 0 1 2 3 4 5 6 7 8 9 10 11

MEAL PLANNER * MONTH ________ YR ____

DAY 22: **MON TUES WED THU FRI SAT SUN** Cal Fat Pro Carbs

B ____________________

L ____________________

S ____________________

D ____________________

DAY 23: **MON TUES WED THU FRI SAT SUN** Cal Fat Pro Carbs

B ____________________

L ____________________

S ____________________

D ____________________

DAY 24: **MON TUES WED THU FRI SAT SUN** Cal Fat Pro Carbs

B ____________________

L ____________________

S ____________________

D ____________________

DAY 25: **MON TUES WED THU FRI SAT SUN** Cal Fat Pro Carbs

B ____________________

L ____________________

S ____________________

D ____________________

DAY 26: **MON TUES WED THU FRI SAT SUN** Cal Fat Pro Carbs

B ____________________

L ____________________

S ____________________

D ____________________

DAY 27: **MON TUES WED THU FRI SAT SUN** Cal Fat Pro Carbs

B ____________________

L ____________________

S ____________________

D ____________________

DAY 28: **MON TUES WED THU FRI SAT SUN** Cal Fat Pro Carbs

B ____________________

L ____________________

S ____________________

D ____________________

DAY 22: **MON TUES WED THU FRI SAT SUN** *Time* *Calories Burned*

Exercise ______

Water ______ Steps ______

Sleep ______ Weight ______

Stress Level 0 1 2 3 4 5 6 7 8 9 10 11

DAY 23: **MON TUES WED THU FRI SAT SUN** *Time* *Calories Burned*

Exercise ______

Water ______ Steps ______

Sleep ______ Weight ______

Stress Level 0 1 2 3 4 5 6 7 8 9 10 11

DAY 24: **MON TUES WED THU FRI SAT SUN** *Time* *Calories Burned*

Exercise ______

Water ______ Steps ______

Sleep ______ Weight ______

Stress Level 0 1 2 3 4 5 6 7 8 9 10 11

DAY 25: **MON TUES WED THU FRI SAT SUN** *Time* *Calories Burned*

Exercise ______

Water ______ Steps ______

Sleep ______ Weight ______

Stress Level 0 1 2 3 4 5 6 7 8 9 10 11

DAY 26: **MON TUES WED THU FRI SAT SUN** *Time* *Calories Burned*

Exercise ______

Water ______ Steps ______

Sleep ______ Weight ______

Stress Level 0 1 2 3 4 5 6 7 8 9 10 11

DAY 27: **MON TUES WED THU FRI SAT SUN** *Time* *Calories Burned*

Exercise ______

Water ______ Steps ______

Sleep ______ Weight ______

Stress Level 0 1 2 3 4 5 6 7 8 9 10 11

DAY 28: **MON TUES WED THU FRI SAT SUN** *Time* *Calories Burned*

Exercise ______

Water ______ Steps ______

Sleep ______ Weight ______

Stress Level 0 1 2 3 4 5 6 7 8 9 10 11

MEAL PLANNER * MONTH ________ YR ____

DAY 29: **MON TUES WED THU FRI SAT SUN** Cal Fat Pro Carbs

B ____________________

L ____________________

S ____________________

D ____________________

DAY 30: **MON TUES WED THU FRI SAT SUN** Cal Fat Pro Carbs

B ____________________

L ____________________

S ____________________

D ____________________

DAY 31: **MON TUES WED THU FRI SAT SUN** Cal Fat Pro Carbs

B ____________________

L ____________________

S ____________________

D ____________________

GOALS

	Achieved Y	Achieved N
1. ____________________	☐	☐
2. ____________________	☐	☐
3. ____________________	☐	☐
4. ____________________	☐	☐
5. ____________________	☐	☐

End of Month Results

Weight

Blood Pressure

Resting Heart Rate

DAY 29: **MON TUES WED THU FRI SAT SUN** *Time* *Calories Burned*

Exercise ______________________________

Water ______________ Steps ______________

Sleep ______________ Weight ______________

Stress Level 0 1 2 3 4 5 6 7 8 9 10 11

DAY 30: **MON TUES WED THU FRI SAT SUN** *Time* *Calories Burned*

Exercise ______________________________

Water ______________ Steps ______________

Sleep ______________ Weight ______________

Stress Level 0 1 2 3 4 5 6 7 8 9 10 11

DAY 31: **MON TUES WED THU FRI SAT SUN** *Time* *Calories Burned*

Exercise ______________________________

Water ______________ Steps ______________

Sleep ______________ Weight ______________

Stress Level 0 1 2 3 4 5 6 7 8 9 10 11

STRESSORS

	Resolved Y	Resolved N
1. ______________	☐	☐
2. ______________	☐	☐
3. ______________	☐	☐
4. ______________	☐	☐
5. ______________	☐	☐

of Successful Days

Count all the days this month you achieved your own health goals.

Exercise ○ Water ○ Steps ○ Sleep ○ Weight ○

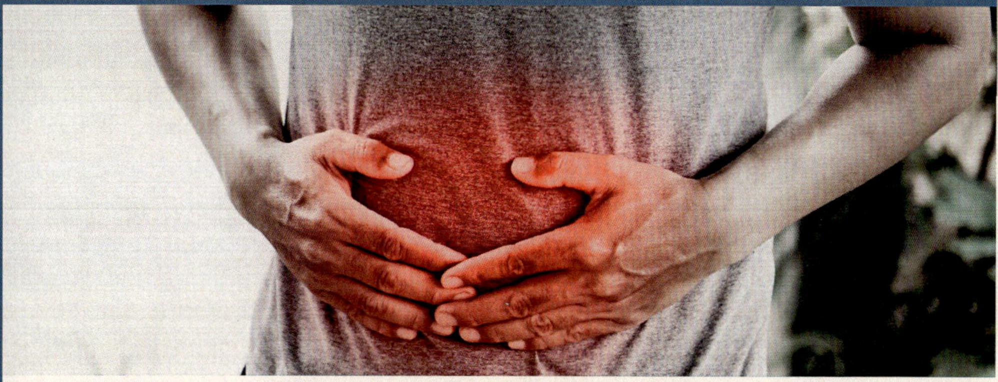

8. GASTRO

Pancreas, Stomach, Small Intestine, Liver
Diabetes, Large Intestine, Colon, Gall Bladder

Issues in the digestive system are related to repressed anger, storing pain, constant worry and needs unmet. The food we eat, and the foods we combine together, make our system work for us or against us. Emotional eating makes us crave unhealthy food, which is a form of self-destruction. We use sugar and fatty food to make up for vitamin deficiencies in our brains, caused by hormonal imbalances. This comes from a gut biome that is under attack. Our gut is the second brain. The more we know, the less we depend on food to pacify us.

Set some goals for the month, and at the end, we will reflect on your progress. You can track your meals, exercise, appointments, and weight goals. Set some spiritual goals too.

GOALS

1. ______________________________
2. ______________________________
3. ______________________________
4. ______________________________
5. ______________________________

"Do you not understand that everything that goes into the mouth passes into the stomach, and is eliminated?"
Matthew 15:17

Monthly Affirmation:

"I am capable of meeting my own needs."

Exercise: *Each day, ask yourself, 'What do I need?" If you can, feel empowered to do it for yourself.*

FOODS to Improve Gastro Health:

- **Beans:** Black-eyed Peas, Miso
- **Fat:** Eggs, Cultured Yogurt, Kefir, Olives, Coconut Oil
- **Fruit:** Berries, Bananas, Figs, Pomegranate, Peach, Cucumber
- **Herb:** Rooibos, Peppermint, Basil, Cilantro, Oregano, Wormwood
- **Protein:** Wild-caught fish
- **Nuts:** Almonds, Cashews, Macadamia Nut, Walnuts
- **Root:** Shallots, Onions, Ginger
- **Vegetables:** Kelp, Kale, Zucchini, Sauerkraut Dandelion, Asparagus
- **Vitamins:** A, B1, B3, B6, B12, C, D, Biotin, L-Glutamine, Probiotics
- **Grains:** Millet, Quinoa, Barley

JUICE to Improve Gastro Health:

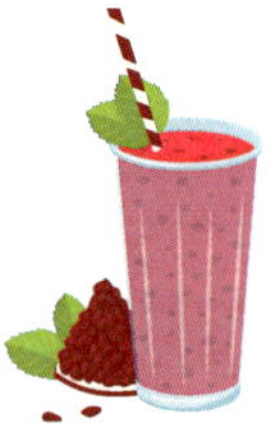

Pomegranate Peach Strawberry

Contact Vandene:
for Local South Florida Delivery
ordersmavis@gmail.com

M.A.V.I.S
Health Drinks

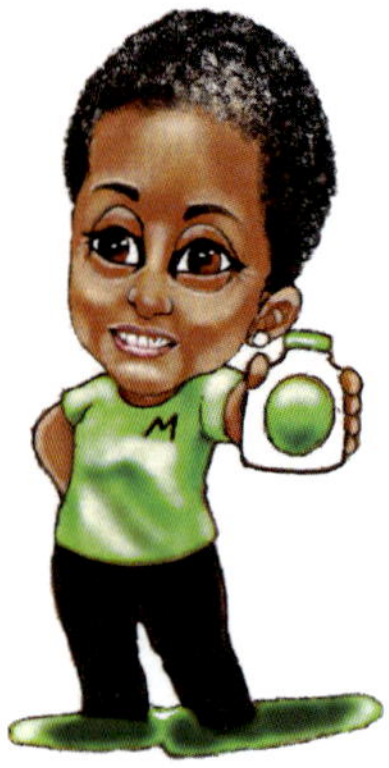

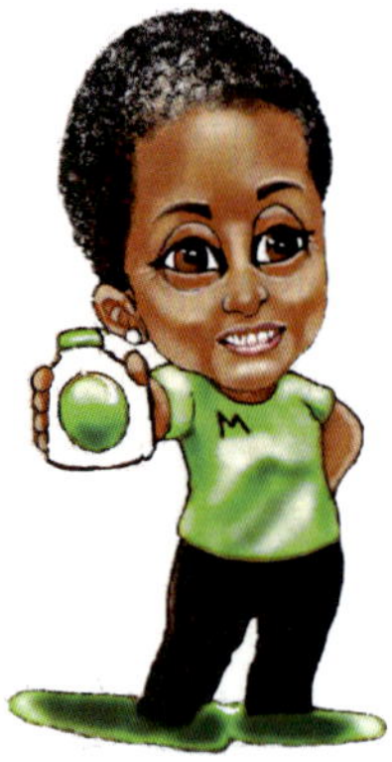

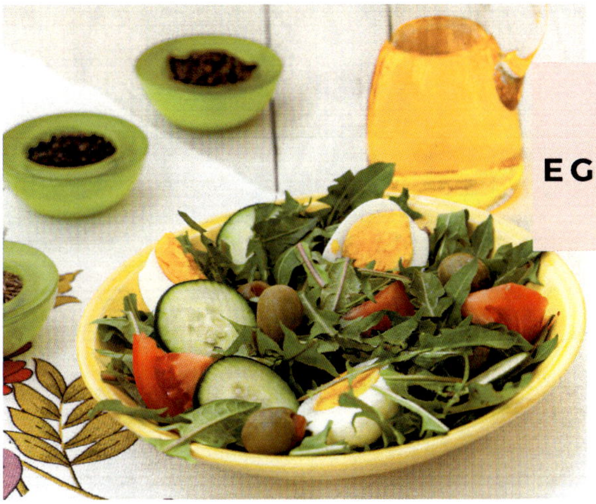

DANDELION W/
EGGS, OLIVES, CUCUMBER

YIELDS 2 SERVINGS

TOTAL TIME: 10 MINS

2 - cups of Dandelion greens
2 - hard-boiled eggs
1 - tsp of Coconut Oil
1 - tsp of Olive Oil
1 - tsp of Lime Juice
1 - cup of Green Olives
1 - sliced Tomato
1 - sliced Cucumber
1/2 - Shallot - finely chopped

DIRECTIONS:

- Whisk Coconut oil and Olive Oil with lime juice in a bowl
- Add dandelion, shallots, cucumber, tomato, olives and toss in dressing
- Cut hard boiled eggs in half
- Serve salad with eggs
- Add mandarin oranges (Optional)

Medical Appointments

Date/Time | Office

____

____

____

____

MEAL PLANNER * MONTH ________ YR ______

DAY 1: **MON TUES WED THU FRI SAT SUN** Cal Fat Pro Carbs

B ____________________

L ____________________

S ____________________

D ____________________

DAY 2: **MON TUES WED THU FRI SAT SUN** Cal Fat Pro Carbs

B ____________________

L ____________________

S ____________________

D ____________________

DAY 3: **MON TUES WED THU FRI SAT SUN** Cal Fat Pro Carbs

B ____________________

L ____________________

S ____________________

D ____________________

DAY 4: **MON TUES WED THU FRI SAT SUN** Cal Fat Pro Carbs

B ____________________

L ____________________

S ____________________

D ____________________

DAY 5: **MON TUES WED THU FRI SAT SUN** Cal Fat Pro Carbs

B ____________________

L ____________________

S ____________________

D ____________________

DAY 6: **MON TUES WED THU FRI SAT SUN** Cal Fat Pro Carbs

B ____________________

L ____________________

S ____________________

D ____________________

DAY 7: **MON TUES WED THU FRI SAT SUN** Cal Fat Pro Carbs

B ____________________

L ____________________

S ____________________

D ____________________

DAY 1: **MON TUES WED THU FRI SAT SUN** *Time* *Calories Burned*

Exercise ______

Water ______ Steps ______

Sleep ______ Weight ______

Stress Level 0 1 2 3 4 5 6 7 8 9 10 11

DAY 2: **MON TUES WED THU FRI SAT SUN** *Time* *Calories Burned*

Exercise ______

Water ______ Steps ______

Sleep ______ Weight ______

Stress Level 0 1 2 3 4 5 6 7 8 9 10 11

DAY 3: **MON TUES WED THU FRI SAT SUN** *Time* *Calories Burned*

Exercise ______

Water ______ Steps ______

Sleep ______ Weight ______

Stress Level 0 1 2 3 4 5 6 7 8 9 10 11

DAY 4: **MON TUES WED THU FRI SAT SUN** *Time* *Calories Burned*

Exercise ______

Water ______ Steps ______

Sleep ______ Weight ______

Stress Level 0 1 2 3 4 5 6 7 8 9 10 11

DAY 5: **MON TUES WED THU FRI SAT SUN** *Time* *Calories Burned*

Exercise ______

Water ______ Steps ______

Sleep ______ Weight ______

Stress Level 0 1 2 3 4 5 6 7 8 9 10 11

DAY 6: **MON TUES WED THU FRI SAT SUN** *Time* *Calories Burned*

Exercise ______

Water ______ Steps ______

Sleep ______ Weight ______

Stress Level 0 1 2 3 4 5 6 7 8 9 10 11

DAY 7: **MON TUES WED THU FRI SAT SUN** *Time* *Calories Burned*

Exercise ______

Water ______ Steps ______

Sleep ______ Weight ______

Stress Level 0 1 2 3 4 5 6 7 8 9 10 11

MEAL PLANNER * MONTH ______ YR ____

DAY 8: **MON TUES WED THU FRI SAT SUN** Cal Fat Pro Carbs

B ____________________

L ____________________

S ____________________

D ____________________

DAY 9: **MON TUES WED THU FRI SAT SUN** Cal Fat Pro Carbs

B ____________________

L ____________________

S ____________________

D ____________________

DAY 10: **MON TUES WED THU FRI SAT SUN** Cal Fat Pro Carbs

B ____________________

L ____________________

S ____________________

D ____________________

DAY 11: **MON TUES WED THU FRI SAT SUN** Cal Fat Pro Carbs

B ____________________

L ____________________

S ____________________

D ____________________

DAY 12: **MON TUES WED THU FRI SAT SUN** Cal Fat Pro Carbs

B ____________________

L ____________________

S ____________________

D ____________________

DAY 13: **MON TUES WED THU FRI SAT SUN** Cal Fat Pro Carbs

B ____________________

L ____________________

S ____________________

D ____________________

DAY 14: **MON TUES WED THU FRI SAT SUN** Cal Fat Pro Carbs

B ____________________

L ____________________

S ____________________

D ____________________

DAY 8: **MON TUES WED THU FRI SAT SUN** *Time* *Calories Burned*

Exercise ____________________
Water ____________ Steps ____________
Sleep ____________ Weight ____________
Stress Level 0 1 2 3 4 5 6 7 8 9 10 11

DAY 9: **MON TUES WED THU FRI SAT SUN** *Time* *Calories Burned*

Exercise ____________________
Water ____________ Steps ____________
Sleep ____________ Weight ____________
Stress Level 0 1 2 3 4 5 6 7 8 9 10 11

DAY 10: **MON TUES WED THU FRI SAT SUN** *Time* *Calories Burned*

Exercise ____________________
Water ____________ Steps ____________
Sleep ____________ Weight ____________
Stress Level 0 1 2 3 4 5 6 7 8 9 10 11

DAY 11: **MON TUES WED THU FRI SAT SUN** *Time* *Calories Burned*

Exercise ____________________
Water ____________ Steps ____________
Sleep ____________ Weight ____________
Stress Level 0 1 2 3 4 5 6 7 8 9 10 11

DAY 12: **MON TUES WED THU FRI SAT SUN** *Time* *Calories Burned*

Exercise ____________________
Water ____________ Steps ____________
Sleep ____________ Weight ____________
Stress Level 0 1 2 3 4 5 6 7 8 9 10 11

DAY 13: **MON TUES WED THU FRI SAT SUN** *Time* *Calories Burned*

Exercise ____________________
Water ____________ Steps ____________
Sleep ____________ Weight ____________
Stress Level 0 1 2 3 4 5 6 7 8 9 10 11

DAY 14: **MON TUES WED THU FRI SAT SUN** *Time* *Calories Burned*

Exercise ____________________
Water ____________ Steps ____________
Sleep ____________ Weight ____________
Stress Level 0 1 2 3 4 5 6 7 8 9 10 11

MEAL PLANNER * MONTH ______ YR ______

DAY 15: **MON TUES WED THU FRI SAT SUN** Cal Fat Pro Carbs

B ____________________

L ____________________

S ____________________

D ____________________

DAY 16: **MON TUES WED THU FRI SAT SUN** Cal Fat Pro Carbs

B ____________________

L ____________________

S ____________________

D ____________________

DAY 17: **MON TUES WED THU FRI SAT SUN** Cal Fat Pro Carbs

B ____________________

L ____________________

S ____________________

D ____________________

DAY 18: **MON TUES WED THU FRI SAT SUN** Cal Fat Pro Carbs

B ____________________

L ____________________

S ____________________

D ____________________

DAY 19: **MON TUES WED THU FRI SAT SUN** Cal Fat Pro Carbs

B ____________________

L ____________________

S ____________________

D ____________________

DAY 20: **MON TUES WED THU FRI SAT SUN** Cal Fat Pro Carbs

B ____________________

L ____________________

S ____________________

D ____________________

DAY 21: **MON TUES WED THU FRI SAT SUN** Cal Fat Pro Carbs

B ____________________

L ____________________

S ____________________

D ____________________

DAY 15: **MON TUES WED THU FRI SAT SUN** *Time* *Calories Burned*

Exercise ______________________________

Water ____________ Steps ____________

Sleep ____________ Weight ____________

Stress Level 0 1 2 3 4 5 6 7 8 9 10 11

DAY 16: **MON TUES WED THU FRI SAT SUN** *Time* *Calories Burned*

Exercise ______________________________

Water ____________ Steps ____________

Sleep ____________ Weight ____________

Stress Level 0 1 2 3 4 5 6 7 8 9 10 11

DAY 17: **MON TUES WED THU FRI SAT SUN** *Time* *Calories Burned*

Exercise ______________________________

Water ____________ Steps ____________

Sleep ____________ Weight ____________

Stress Level 0 1 2 3 4 5 6 7 8 9 10 11

DAY 18: **MON TUES WED THU FRI SAT SUN** *Time* *Calories Burned*

Exercise ______________________________

Water ____________ Steps ____________

Sleep ____________ Weight ____________

Stress Level 0 1 2 3 4 5 6 7 8 9 10 11

DAY 19: **MON TUES WED THU FRI SAT SUN** *Time* *Calories Burned*

Exercise ______________________________

Water ____________ Steps ____________

Sleep ____________ Weight ____________

Stress Level 0 1 2 3 4 5 6 7 8 9 10 11

DAY 20: **MON TUES WED THU FRI SAT SUN** *Time* *Calories Burned*

Exercise ______________________________

Water ____________ Steps ____________

Sleep ____________ Weight ____________

Stress Level 0 1 2 3 4 5 6 7 8 9 10 11

DAY 21: **MON TUES WED THU FRI SAT SUN** *Time* *Calories Burned*

Exercise ______________________________

Water ____________ Steps ____________

Sleep ____________ Weight ____________

Stress Level 0 1 2 3 4 5 6 7 8 9 10 11

MEAL PLANNER * MONTH ________ YR ____

DAY 22: **MON TUES WED THU FRI SAT SUN** Cal Fat Pro Carbs

B ____________________

L ____________________

S ____________________

D ____________________

DAY 23: **MON TUES WED THU FRI SAT SUN** Cal Fat Pro Carbs

B ____________________

L ____________________

S ____________________

D ____________________

DAY 24: **MON TUES WED THU FRI SAT SUN** Cal Fat Pro Carbs

B ____________________

L ____________________

S ____________________

D ____________________

DAY 25: **MON TUES WED THU FRI SAT SUN** Cal Fat Pro Carbs

B ____________________

L ____________________

S ____________________

D ____________________

DAY 26: **MON TUES WED THU FRI SAT SUN** Cal Fat Pro Carbs

B ____________________

L ____________________

S ____________________

D ____________________

DAY 27: **MON TUES WED THU FRI SAT SUN** Cal Fat Pro Carbs

B ____________________

L ____________________

S ____________________

D ____________________

DAY 28: **MON TUES WED THU FRI SAT SUN** Cal Fat Pro Carbs

B ____________________

L ____________________

S ____________________

D ____________________

DAY 22: **MON TUES WED THU FRI SAT SUN** *Time* *Calories Burned*

Exercise ______
Water ______ Steps ______
Sleep ______ Weight ______
Stress Level 0 1 2 3 4 5 6 7 8 9 10 11

DAY 23: **MON TUES WED THU FRI SAT SUN** *Time* *Calories Burned*

Exercise ______
Water ______ Steps ______
Sleep ______ Weight ______
Stress Level 0 1 2 3 4 5 6 7 8 9 10 11

DAY 24: **MON TUES WED THU FRI SAT SUN** *Time* *Calories Burned*

Exercise ______
Water ______ Steps ______
Sleep ______ Weight ______
Stress Level 0 1 2 3 4 5 6 7 8 9 10 11

DAY 25: **MON TUES WED THU FRI SAT SUN** *Time* *Calories Burned*

Exercise ______
Water ______ Steps ______
Sleep ______ Weight ______
Stress Level 0 1 2 3 4 5 6 7 8 9 10 11

DAY 26: **MON TUES WED THU FRI SAT SUN** *Time* *Calories Burned*

Exercise ______
Water ______ Steps ______
Sleep ______ Weight ______
Stress Level 0 1 2 3 4 5 6 7 8 9 10 11

DAY 27: **MON TUES WED THU FRI SAT SUN** *Time* *Calories Burned*

Exercise ______
Water ______ Steps ______
Sleep ______ Weight ______
Stress Level 0 1 2 3 4 5 6 7 8 9 10 11

DAY 28: **MON TUES WED THU FRI SAT SUN** *Time* *Calories Burned*

Exercise ______
Water ______ Steps ______
Sleep ______ Weight ______
Stress Level 0 1 2 3 4 5 6 7 8 9 10 11

MEAL PLANNER * MONTH ________ YR ____

DAY 29: MON TUES WED THU FRI SAT SUN Cal Fat Pro Carbs

B ______

L ______

S ______

D ______

DAY 30: MON TUES WED THU FRI SAT SUN Cal Fat Pro Carbs

B ______

L ______

S ______

D ______

DAY 31: MON TUES WED THU FRI SAT SUN Cal Fat Pro Carbs

B ______

L ______

S ______

D ______

GOALS

	Achieved Y	N
1. ______	☐	☐
2. ______	☐	☐
3. ______	☐	☐
4. ______	☐	☐
5. ______	☐	☐

End of Month Results

Weight

Blood Pressure

Resting Heart Rate

DAY 29: **MON TUES WED THU FRI SAT SUN** *Time* *Calories Burned*

Exercise ______________________________

Water ______________ Steps ______________

Sleep ______________ Weight ______________

Stress Level 0 1 2 3 4 5 6 7 8 9 10 11

DAY 30: **MON TUES WED THU FRI SAT SUN** *Time* *Calories Burned*

Exercise ______________________________

Water ______________ Steps ______________

Sleep ______________ Weight ______________

Stress Level 0 1 2 3 4 5 6 7 8 9 10 11

DAY 31: **MON TUES WED THU FRI SAT SUN** *Time* *Calories Burned*

Exercise ______________________________

Water ______________ Steps ______________

Sleep ______________ Weight ______________

Stress Level 0 1 2 3 4 5 6 7 8 9 10 11

STRESSORS

	Resolved Y	Resolved N
1. ______________	☐	☐
2. ______________	☐	☐
3. ______________	☐	☐
4. ______________	☐	☐
5. ______________	☐	☐

of Successful Days

Count all the days this month you achieved your own health goals.

Exercise Water Steps Sleep Weight

ACTIVITY PLANNER * MONTH ________ YR ____

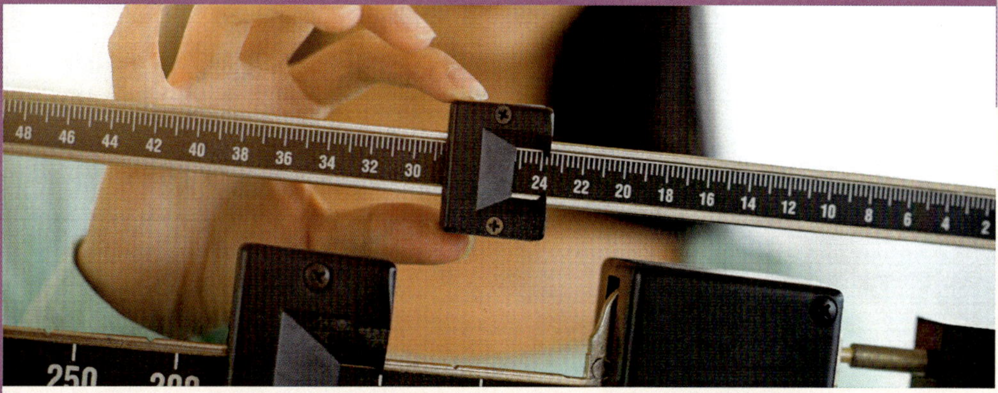

9. METABOLISM

Weight, Eating Disorders, Food Addiction
Obesity, Candida

Food addiction is not about food. The spiritual cause of food addiction is lack of happiness. The fat gained from emotional eating, pads the body for protection. When we feel unsafe, unable to trust others, we crave security in the form of a quick fix. We can't endure the pain of discomfort, because we have endured it for too long, with no relief. We have already learned that no one is coming to save us from our pain, so we self-medicate with food. Our metabolism responds by creating a dis-order. There are organisms in our body that benefit from this disorder, such as Candida. Candida is likely the root cause of depression.

Set some goals for the month, and at the end, we will reflect on your progress. You can track your meals, exercise, appointments, and weight goals. Set some spiritual goals too.

GOALS

1. ________________________________
2. ________________________________
3. ________________________________
4. ________________________________
5. ________________________________

> *"They shall hunger no more, neither thirst any more; neither shall the sun light on them, nor any heat. For the Lamb which is in the midst of the throne shall feed them, and shall lead them unto living fountains of waters: and God shall wipe away all tears from their eyes."*
>
> *Revelations 7:16-17*

Monthly Affirmation:

"I am safe in my mind, body, and soul."

Exercise: *Become aware of your triggers. Who is the one responsible for how you respond? Know thyself.*

FOODS to Improve Metabolism Health:

- **Beans:** Dried Red Beans, Lentils, Black, Chickpeas
- Fat: Hemp Oil, Flaxseed Oil, Greek Yogurt
- Fruit: Tangerine, Limes, Lemons, Blackberries, Red Grapefruit
- Herb: Fenugreek, Ginseng, Turmeric, Oregano
- **Protein:** Salmon, Tempeh, Tofu, Tuna, Halibut
- **Nuts:** Almonds, Walnuts, Pecans, Hazelnuts
- Root: Cinnamon, Garlic, Ginger
- **Vegetables:** Hot Peppers, Cayenne, Broccoli, Asparagus
- **Vitamins:** Iron, Zinc, Selenium
- Grains: Brown Rice, Quinoa

JUICE to Improve Metabolism Health:

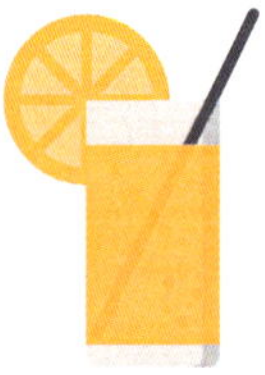

Lemon
Ginger
Cayenne

Contact Vandene:
for Local South Florida Delivery
ordersmavis@gmail.com

M.A.V.I.S
Health Drinks

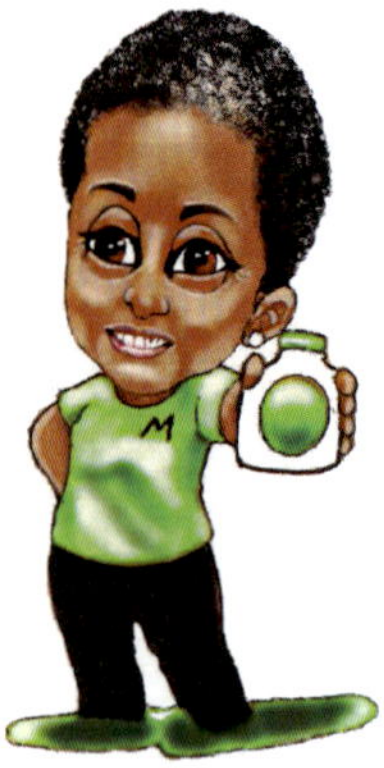

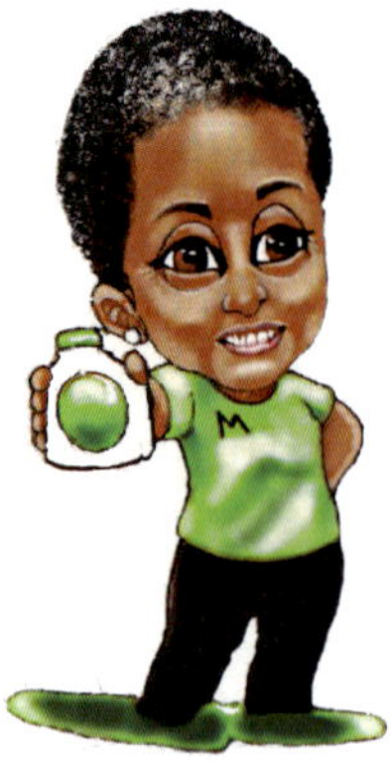

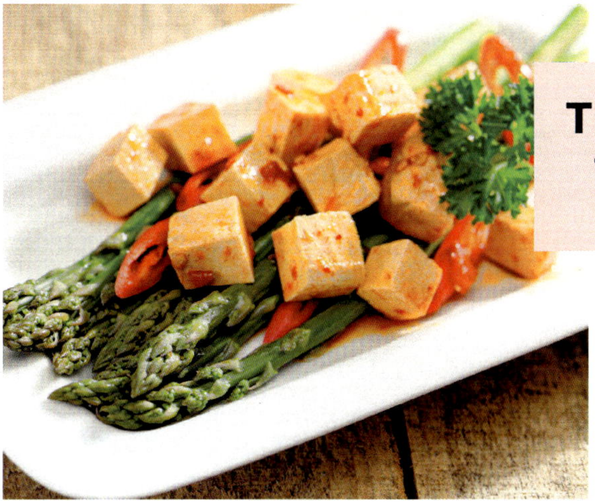

TANGERINE MISO TOFU W/ ASPARAGUS

YIELDS 2 SERVINGS

TOTAL TIME: 35 MINS

1 - 14 oz. extra-firm tofu
2 - tbsp red miso paste
4 - tsp of Sesame Oil
1 - pound of Asparagus
3 - tbsps of Fresh Basil, chopped
1 - tsp of tangerine zest
1 - Tangerine (Juiced)
1 - dash of sea salt
2 - cloves of Garlic
1 - cup of brown rice
2 - tbsp of Tamari or soy sauce
2 - Scallions, chopped
2 - tbsp Turbinado Sugar

DIRECTIONS:

- Cook brown rice as directed
- Preheat oven to 400 degrees F
- Drain tofu, pat dry, and cut into 1 inch cubes
- In a bowl, add garlic, tangerine juice, sugar, zest, salt, Tamari, and miso paste. Whisk.
- Add tofu cubes to coat, save some sauce
- Place tofu flat on a greased baking sheet
- Bake for 15 minutes
- Toss asparagus in sauce, save some sauce
- Add asparagus to baking sheet and bake with tofu for 10 more minutes
- Add chopped basil and scallions to sauce
- Toss separately tofu, then asparagus in bowl
- Serve with brown rice

Medical Appointments

Date/Time	Office

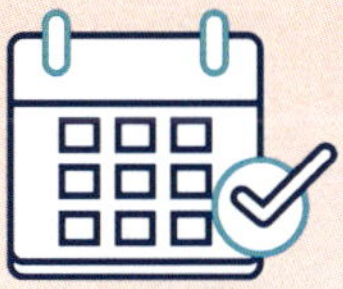

MEAL PLANNER * MONTH ________ YR ____

DAY 1: **MON TUES WED THU FRI SAT SUN** Cal Fat Pro Carbs

B ______
L ______
S ______
D ______

DAY 2: **MON TUES WED THU FRI SAT SUN** Cal Fat Pro Carbs

B ______
L ______
S ______
D ______

DAY 3: **MON TUES WED THU FRI SAT SUN** Cal Fat Pro Carbs

B ______
L ______
S ______
D ______

DAY 4: **MON TUES WED THU FRI SAT SUN** Cal Fat Pro Carbs

B ______
L ______
S ______
D ______

DAY 5: **MON TUES WED THU FRI SAT SUN** Cal Fat Pro Carbs

B ______
L ______
S ______
D ______

DAY 6: **MON TUES WED THU FRI SAT SUN** Cal Fat Pro Carbs

B ______
L ______
S ______
D ______

DAY 7: **MON TUES WED THU FRI SAT SUN** Cal Fat Pro Carbs

B ______
L ______
S ______
D ______

DAY 1: **MON TUES WED THU FRI SAT SUN** *Time* *Calories Burned*

Exercise ______

Water ______ Steps ______

Sleep ______ Weight ______

Stress Level 0 1 2 3 4 5 6 7 8 9 10 11

DAY 2: **MON TUES WED THU FRI SAT SUN** *Time* *Calories Burned*

Exercise ______

Water ______ Steps ______

Sleep ______ Weight ______

Stress Level 0 1 2 3 4 5 6 7 8 9 10 11

DAY 3: **MON TUES WED THU FRI SAT SUN** *Time* *Calories Burned*

Exercise ______

Water ______ Steps ______

Sleep ______ Weight ______

Stress Level 0 1 2 3 4 5 6 7 8 9 10 11

DAY 4: **MON TUES WED THU FRI SAT SUN** *Time* *Calories Burned*

Exercise ______

Water ______ Steps ______

Sleep ______ Weight ______

Stress Level 0 1 2 3 4 5 6 7 8 9 10 11

DAY 5: **MON TUES WED THU FRI SAT SUN** *Time* *Calories Burned*

Exercise ______

Water ______ Steps ______

Sleep ______ Weight ______

Stress Level 0 1 2 3 4 5 6 7 8 9 10 11

DAY 6: **MON TUES WED THU FRI SAT SUN** *Time* *Calories Burned*

Exercise ______

Water ______ Steps ______

Sleep ______ Weight ______

Stress Level 0 1 2 3 4 5 6 7 8 9 10 11

DAY 7: **MON TUES WED THU FRI SAT SUN** *Time* *Calories Burned*

Exercise ______

Water ______ Steps ______

Sleep ______ Weight ______

Stress Level 0 1 2 3 4 5 6 7 8 9 10 11

MEAL PLANNER * MONTH ________ YR ____

DAY 8: **MON TUES WED THU FRI SAT SUN** Cal Fat Pro Carbs

B ____________________
L ____________________
S ____________________
D ____________________

DAY 9: **MON TUES WED THU FRI SAT SUN** Cal Fat Pro Carbs

B ____________________
L ____________________
S ____________________
D ____________________

DAY 10: **MON TUES WED THU FRI SAT SUN** Cal Fat Pro Carbs

B ____________________
L ____________________
S ____________________
D ____________________

DAY 11: **MON TUES WED THU FRI SAT SUN** Cal Fat Pro Carbs

B ____________________
L ____________________
S ____________________
D ____________________

DAY 12: **MON TUES WED THU FRI SAT SUN** Cal Fat Pro Carbs

B ____________________
L ____________________
S ____________________
D ____________________

DAY 13: **MON TUES WED THU FRI SAT SUN** Cal Fat Pro Carbs

B ____________________
L ____________________
S ____________________
D ____________________

DAY 14: **MON TUES WED THU FRI SAT SUN** Cal Fat Pro Carbs

B ____________________
L ____________________
S ____________________
D ____________________

DAY 8: **MON TUES WED THU FRI SAT SUN** *Time* *Calories Burned*

Exercise ______

Water ______ Steps ______

Sleep ______ Weight ______

Stress Level 0 1 2 3 4 5 6 7 8 9 10 11

DAY 9: **MON TUES WED THU FRI SAT SUN** *Time* *Calories Burned*

Exercise ______

Water ______ Steps ______

Sleep ______ Weight ______

Stress Level 0 1 2 3 4 5 6 7 8 9 10 11

DAY 10: **MON TUES WED THU FRI SAT SUN** *Time* *Calories Burned*

Exercise ______

Water ______ Steps ______

Sleep ______ Weight ______

Stress Level 0 1 2 3 4 5 6 7 8 9 10 11

DAY 11: **MON TUES WED THU FRI SAT SUN** *Time* *Calories Burned*

Exercise ______

Water ______ Steps ______

Sleep ______ Weight ______

Stress Level 0 1 2 3 4 5 6 7 8 9 10 11

DAY 12: **MON TUES WED THU FRI SAT SUN** *Time* *Calories Burned*

Exercise ______

Water ______ Steps ______

Sleep ______ Weight ______

Stress Level 0 1 2 3 4 5 6 7 8 9 10 11

DAY 13: **MON TUES WED THU FRI SAT SUN** *Time* *Calories Burned*

Exercise ______

Water ______ Steps ______

Sleep ______ Weight ______

Stress Level 0 1 2 3 4 5 6 7 8 9 10 11

DAY 14: **MON TUES WED THU FRI SAT SUN** *Time* *Calories Burned*

Exercise ______

Water ______ Steps ______

Sleep ______ Weight ______

Stress Level 0 1 2 3 4 5 6 7 8 9 10 11

DAY 15: **MON TUES WED THU FRI SAT SUN** Cal Fat Pro Carbs

B ____
L ____
S ____
D ____

DAY 16: **MON TUES WED THU FRI SAT SUN** Cal Fat Pro Carbs

B ____
L ____
S ____
D ____

DAY 17: **MON TUES WED THU FRI SAT SUN** Cal Fat Pro Carbs

B ____
L ____
S ____
D ____

DAY 18: **MON TUES WED THU FRI SAT SUN** Cal Fat Pro Carbs

B ____
L ____
S ____
D ____

DAY 19: **MON TUES WED THU FRI SAT SUN** Cal Fat Pro Carbs

B ____
L ____
S ____
D ____

DAY 20: **MON TUES WED THU FRI SAT SUN** Cal Fat Pro Carbs

B ____
L ____
S ____
D ____

DAY 21: **MON TUES WED THU FRI SAT SUN** Cal Fat Pro Carbs

B ____
L ____
S ____
D ____

DAY 15: **MON TUES WED THU FRI SAT SUN** *Time* *Calories Burned*

Exercise ______________________________

Water ______________ Steps ______________

Sleep ______________ Weight ______________

Stress Level 0 1 2 3 4 5 6 7 8 9 10 11

DAY 16: **MON TUES WED THU FRI SAT SUN** *Time* *Calories Burned*

Exercise ______________________________

Water ______________ Steps ______________

Sleep ______________ Weight ______________

Stress Level 0 1 2 3 4 5 6 7 8 9 10 11

DAY 17: **MON TUES WED THU FRI SAT SUN** *Time* *Calories Burned*

Exercise ______________________________

Water ______________ Steps ______________

Sleep ______________ Weight ______________

Stress Level 0 1 2 3 4 5 6 7 8 9 10 11

DAY 18: **MON TUES WED THU FRI SAT SUN** *Time* *Calories Burned*

Exercise ______________________________

Water ______________ Steps ______________

Sleep ______________ Weight ______________

Stress Level 0 1 2 3 4 5 6 7 8 9 10 11

DAY 19: **MON TUES WED THU FRI SAT SUN** *Time* *Calories Burned*

Exercise ______________________________

Water ______________ Steps ______________

Sleep ______________ Weight ______________

Stress Level 0 1 2 3 4 5 6 7 8 9 10 11

DAY 20: **MON TUES WED THU FRI SAT SUN** *Time* *Calories Burned*

Exercise ______________________________

Water ______________ Steps ______________

Sleep ______________ Weight ______________

Stress Level 0 1 2 3 4 5 6 7 8 9 10 11

DAY 21: **MON TUES WED THU FRI SAT SUN** *Time* *Calories Burned*

Exercise ______________________________

Water ______________ Steps ______________

Sleep ______________ Weight ______________

Stress Level 0 1 2 3 4 5 6 7 8 9 10 11

MEAL PLANNER * MONTH ______ YR ____

DAY 22: **MON TUES WED THU FRI SAT SUN** Cal Fat Pro Carbs

B ____________________
L ____________________
S ____________________
D ____________________

DAY 23: **MON TUES WED THU FRI SAT SUN** Cal Fat Pro Carbs

B ____________________
L ____________________
S ____________________
D ____________________

DAY 24: **MON TUES WED THU FRI SAT SUN** Cal Fat Pro Carbs

B ____________________
L ____________________
S ____________________
D ____________________

DAY 25: **MON TUES WED THU FRI SAT SUN** Cal Fat Pro Carbs

B ____________________
L ____________________
S ____________________
D ____________________

DAY 26: **MON TUES WED THU FRI SAT SUN** Cal Fat Pro Carbs

B ____________________
L ____________________
S ____________________
D ____________________

DAY 27: **MON TUES WED THU FRI SAT SUN** Cal Fat Pro Carbs

B ____________________
L ____________________
S ____________________
D ____________________

DAY 28: **MON TUES WED THU FRI SAT SUN** Cal Fat Pro Carbs

B ____________________
L ____________________
S ____________________
D ____________________

DAY 22: **MON TUES WED THU FRI SAT SUN** *Time* *Calories Burned*

Exercise ______

Water ______ Steps ______

Sleep ______ Weight ______

Stress Level 0 1 2 3 4 5 6 7 8 9 10 11

DAY 23: **MON TUES WED THU FRI SAT SUN** *Time* *Calories Burned*

Exercise ______

Water ______ Steps ______

Sleep ______ Weight ______

Stress Level 0 1 2 3 4 5 6 7 8 9 10 11

DAY 24: **MON TUES WED THU FRI SAT SUN** *Time* *Calories Burned*

Exercise ______

Water ______ Steps ______

Sleep ______ Weight ______

Stress Level 0 1 2 3 4 5 6 7 8 9 10 11

DAY 25: **MON TUES WED THU FRI SAT SUN** *Time* *Calories Burned*

Exercise ______

Water ______ Steps ______

Sleep ______ Weight ______

Stress Level 0 1 2 3 4 5 6 7 8 9 10 11

DAY 26: **MON TUES WED THU FRI SAT SUN** *Time* *Calories Burned*

Exercise ______

Water ______ Steps ______

Sleep ______ Weight ______

Stress Level 0 1 2 3 4 5 6 7 8 9 10 11

DAY 27: **MON TUES WED THU FRI SAT SUN** *Time* *Calories Burned*

Exercise ______

Water ______ Steps ______

Sleep ______ Weight ______

Stress Level 0 1 2 3 4 5 6 7 8 9 10 11

DAY 28: **MON TUES WED THU FRI SAT SUN** *Time* *Calories Burned*

Exercise ______

Water ______ Steps ______

Sleep ______ Weight ______

Stress Level 0 1 2 3 4 5 6 7 8 9 10 11

MEAL PLANNER * MONTH ________ YR ____

DAY 29: MON TUES WED THU FRI SAT SUN Cal Fat Pro Carbs

B ____________________
L ____________________
S ____________________
D ____________________

DAY 30: MON TUES WED THU FRI SAT SUN Cal Fat Pro Carbs

B ____________________
L ____________________
S ____________________
D ____________________

DAY 31: MON TUES WED THU FRI SAT SUN Cal Fat Pro Carbs

B ____________________
L ____________________
S ____________________
D ____________________

GOALS

Achieved (Y) (N)

1. ____________________ ☐ ☐
2. ____________________ ☐ ☐
3. ____________________ ☐ ☐
4. ____________________ ☐ ☐
5. ____________________ ☐ ☐

End of Month Results

Weight

Blood Pressure

Resting Heart Rate

DAY 29: **MON TUES WED THU FRI SAT SUN** *Time* *Calories Burned*

Exercise ______________________________

Water ______________ Steps ______________

Sleep ______________ Weight ______________

Stress Level 0 1 2 3 4 5 6 7 8 9 10 11

DAY 30: **MON TUES WED THU FRI SAT SUN** *Time* *Calories Burned*

Exercise ______________________________

Water ______________ Steps ______________

Sleep ______________ Weight ______________

Stress Level 0 1 2 3 4 5 6 7 8 9 10 11

DAY 31: **MON TUES WED THU FRI SAT SUN** *Time* *Calories Burned*

Exercise ______________________________

Water ______________ Steps ______________

Sleep ______________ Weight ______________

Stress Level 0 1 2 3 4 5 6 7 8 9 10 11

STRESSORS

	Resolved Y	Resolved N
1. ______________________	☐	☐
2. ______________________	☐	☐
3. ______________________	☐	☐
4. ______________________	☐	☐
5. ______________________	☐	☐

of Successful Days

Count all the days this month you achieved your own health goals.

Exercise ◯ Water ◯ Steps ◯ Sleep ◯ Weight ◯

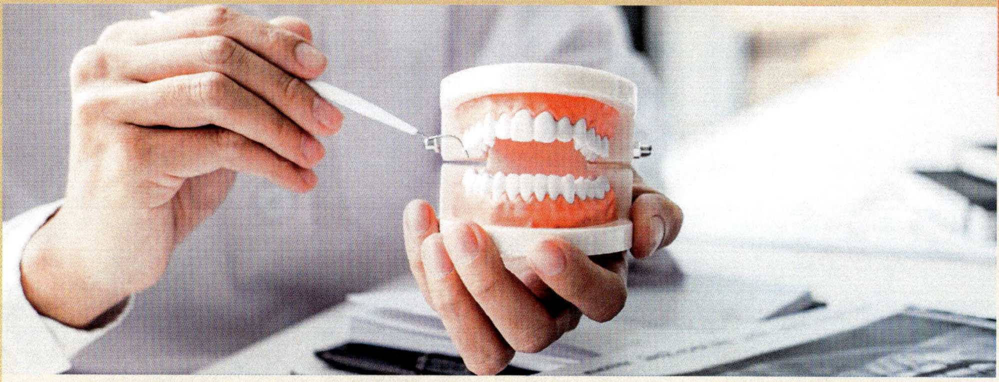

10. DENTAL

Teeth, Gum Tissue, Crown, Enamel, Nerve Root, Bone, Oral Hygiene

When we feel that we can't express ourselves, it can manifest into problems with our teeth, gums, tongue, cavities, or throat. What we speak determines how we are perceived by others. The fear of the perception of others, causes us to hold things inside, to the point of boiling over, then what comes out is mean, cruel and vicious. If we are more expressive with our words, we won't get stuck holding in our emotions, our teeth won't crack, our gums won't recede, and we won't have cavities. Expressing ourselves is a form of self-love.

Set some goals for the month, and at the end, we will reflect on your progress. You can track your meals, exercise, appointments, and weight goals. Set some spiritual goals too.

GOALS

1. ______________________________
2. ______________________________
3. ______________________________
4. ______________________________
5. ______________________________

"Let the words of my mouth, and the meditation of my heart, be acceptable in thy sight, O Lord, my strength, and my redeemer."
Psalms 19:14

Monthly Affirmation:

"I am honest with myself and others."

Exercise: *Tell your story without embellishments. Be as close to your true self as possible. Be Authentic.*

FOODS to Improve Dental Health:

- **Beans:** Green Beans, Snap Peas
- Fat: Yogurt, Eggs, Coconut Oil
- Fruit: Oranges, Apples, Raisins, Kiwi, Strawberries
- Herb: Black Tea, Green Tea, Ginger
- **Protein:** Tofu, Salmon, Chicken
- **Nuts:** Almonds, Cashews
- Root: Raw Carrots, Sweet Potato, Pumpkin
- **Vegetables:** Arugula, Turnip Greens, Celery, Onions, Shiitake Mushrooms
- **Vitamins:** Calcium, D, C, Folate, Manganese
- Grains: Poppy Seeds, Chia Seeds, Sesame Seeds

JUICE to Improve Dental Health:

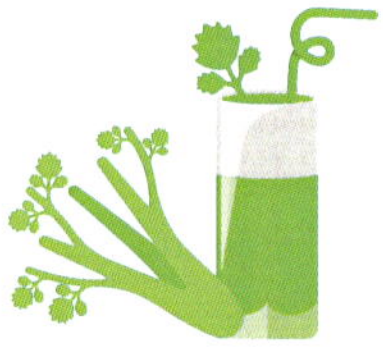

Celery
Apple
Kiwi

Contact Vandene:
for Local South Florida Delivery
ordersmavis@gmail.com

M.A.V.I.S
Health Drinks

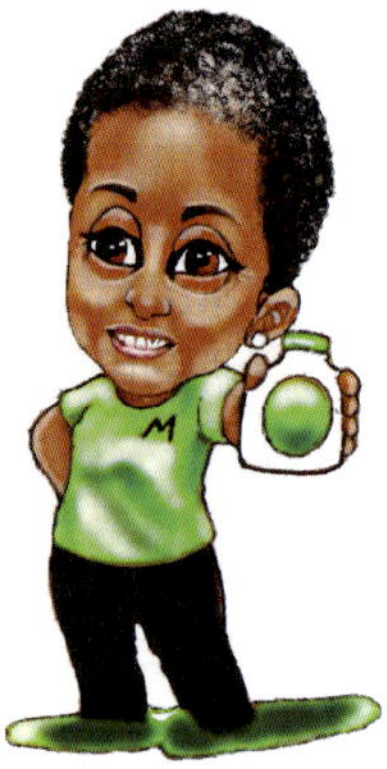

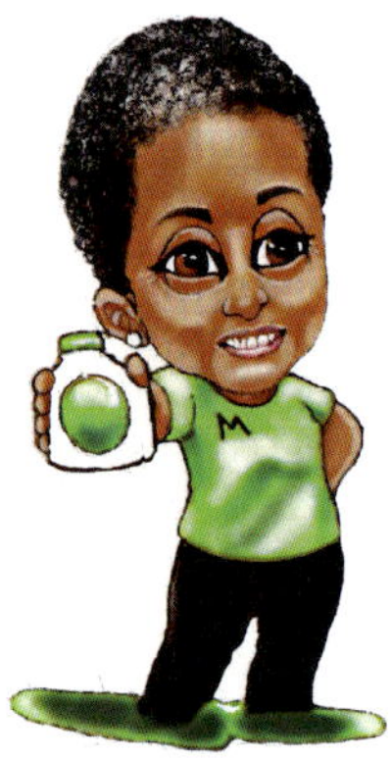

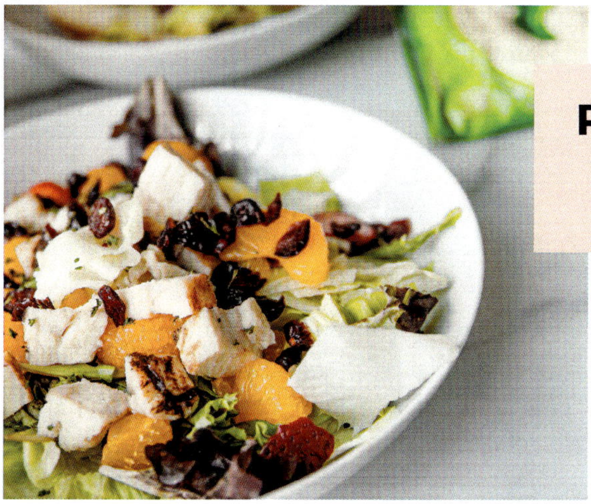

RAISIN ORANGE
SALAD W/ CHICKEN

YIELDS 2 SERVINGS

TOTAL TIME: 10 MINS

1 - 5 oz bag of Spring Mix Salad
2 - Mandarin oranges, peeled
1/4 - cup of Raisins
1/4 - cup of sliced Almonds
1 - cup of Grilled Chicken, diced
3 - tbsps of Fresh Basil, chopped
1/2 - Orange Juice Concentrate (Frozen)
1/4 - cup of Coconut Oil
1 - tbsp of raw Sugar
1 - tsp of Apple Cider Vinegar
1/2 - tbsp of Lemon Juice
1/2 - tsp of Poppy Seeds
1/4 - tsp of Sea Salt

DIRECTIONS:

- Dressing: Mix Coconut Oil, Vinegar, Lemon Juice, Sea Salt, Orange Juice Concentrate, Sugar in a jar. Shake well.
- Top the Spring Mix Salad with Mandarin Oranges, Raisins and Almonds
- Add Grilled Chicken (diced)
- Add Poppy Seeds to dressing.
- Serve Salad with dressing

Medical Appointments

Date/Time Office

____

____

____

____

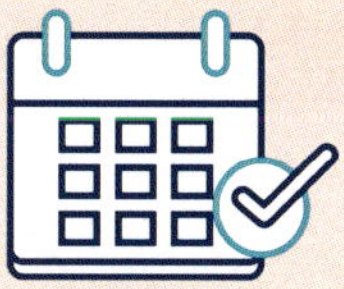

MEAL PLANNER * MONTH ________ YR ____

DAY 1: **MON TUES WED THU FRI SAT SUN** Cal Fat Pro Carbs

B ______________________________

L ______________________________

S ______________________________

D ______________________________

DAY 2: **MON TUES WED THU FRI SAT SUN** Cal Fat Pro Carbs

B ______________________________

L ______________________________

S ______________________________

D ______________________________

DAY 3: **MON TUES WED THU FRI SAT SUN** Cal Fat Pro Carbs

B ______________________________

L ______________________________

S ______________________________

D ______________________________

DAY 4: **MON TUES WED THU FRI SAT SUN** Cal Fat Pro Carbs

B ______________________________

L ______________________________

S ______________________________

D ______________________________

DAY 5: **MON TUES WED THU FRI SAT SUN** Cal Fat Pro Carbs

B ______________________________

L ______________________________

S ______________________________

D ______________________________

DAY 6: **MON TUES WED THU FRI SAT SUN** Cal Fat Pro Carbs

B ______________________________

L ______________________________

S ______________________________

D ______________________________

DAY 7: **MON TUES WED THU FRI SAT SUN** Cal Fat Pro Carbs

B ______________________________

L ______________________________

S ______________________________

D ______________________________

DAY 1: **MON TUES WED THU FRI SAT SUN** *Time* *Calories Burned*

Exercise ______________________________

Water ______________ Steps ______________

Sleep ______________ Weight ______________

Stress Level 0 1 2 3 4 5 6 7 8 9 10 11

DAY 2: **MON TUES WED THU FRI SAT SUN** *Time* *Calories Burned*

Exercise ______________________________

Water ______________ Steps ______________

Sleep ______________ Weight ______________

Stress Level 0 1 2 3 4 5 6 7 8 9 10 11

DAY 3: **MON TUES WED THU FRI SAT SUN** *Time* *Calories Burned*

Exercise ______________________________

Water ______________ Steps ______________

Sleep ______________ Weight ______________

Stress Level 0 1 2 3 4 5 6 7 8 9 10 11

DAY 4: **MON TUES WED THU FRI SAT SUN** *Time* *Calories Burned*

Exercise ______________________________

Water ______________ Steps ______________

Sleep ______________ Weight ______________

Stress Level 0 1 2 3 4 5 6 7 8 9 10 11

DAY 5: **MON TUES WED THU FRI SAT SUN** *Time* *Calories Burned*

Exercise ______________________________

Water ______________ Steps ______________

Sleep ______________ Weight ______________

Stress Level 0 1 2 3 4 5 6 7 8 9 10 11

DAY 6: **MON TUES WED THU FRI SAT SUN** *Time* *Calories Burned*

Exercise ______________________________

Water ______________ Steps ______________

Sleep ______________ Weight ______________

Stress Level 0 1 2 3 4 5 6 7 8 9 10 11

DAY 7: **MON TUES WED THU FRI SAT SUN** *Time* *Calories Burned*

Exercise ______________________________

Water ______________ Steps ______________

Sleep ______________ Weight ______________

Stress Level 0 1 2 3 4 5 6 7 8 9 10 11

MEAL PLANNER * MONTH ________ YR ____

DAY 8: MON TUES WED THU FRI SAT SUN Cal Fat Pro Carbs

B ____

L ____

S ____

D ____

DAY 9: MON TUES WED THU FRI SAT SUN Cal Fat Pro Carbs

B ____

L ____

S ____

D ____

DAY 10: MON TUES WED THU FRI SAT SUN Cal Fat Pro Carbs

B ____

L ____

S ____

D ____

DAY 11: MON TUES WED THU FRI SAT SUN Cal Fat Pro Carbs

B ____

L ____

S ____

D ____

DAY 12: MON TUES WED THU FRI SAT SUN Cal Fat Pro Carbs

B ____

L ____

S ____

D ____

DAY 13: MON TUES WED THU FRI SAT SUN Cal Fat Pro Carbs

B ____

L ____

S ____

D ____

DAY 14: MON TUES WED THU FRI SAT SUN Cal Fat Pro Carbs

B ____

L ____

S ____

D ____

DAY 8: **MON TUES WED THU FRI SAT SUN** *Time* *Calories Burned*

Exercise ______

Water ______ Steps ______

Sleep ______ Weight ______

Stress Level 0 1 2 3 4 5 6 7 8 9 10 11

DAY 9: **MON TUES WED THU FRI SAT SUN** *Time* *Calories Burned*

Exercise ______

Water ______ Steps ______

Sleep ______ Weight ______

Stress Level 0 1 2 3 4 5 6 7 8 9 10 11

DAY 10: **MON TUES WED THU FRI SAT SUN** *Time* *Calories Burned*

Exercise ______

Water ______ Steps ______

Sleep ______ Weight ______

Stress Level 0 1 2 3 4 5 6 7 8 9 10 11

DAY 11: **MON TUES WED THU FRI SAT SUN** *Time* *Calories Burned*

Exercise ______

Water ______ Steps ______

Sleep ______ Weight ______

Stress Level 0 1 2 3 4 5 6 7 8 9 10 11

DAY 12: **MON TUES WED THU FRI SAT SUN** *Time* *Calories Burned*

Exercise ______

Water ______ Steps ______

Sleep ______ Weight ______

Stress Level 0 1 2 3 4 5 6 7 8 9 10 11

DAY 13: **MON TUES WED THU FRI SAT SUN** *Time* *Calories Burned*

Exercise ______

Water ______ Steps ______

Sleep ______ Weight ______

Stress Level 0 1 2 3 4 5 6 7 8 9 10 11

DAY 14: **MON TUES WED THU FRI SAT SUN** *Time* *Calories Burned*

Exercise ______

Water ______ Steps ______

Sleep ______ Weight ______

Stress Level 0 1 2 3 4 5 6 7 8 9 10 11

MEAL PLANNER * MONTH ___ ___ YR ___

DAY 15: **MON TUES WED THU FRI SAT SUN** Cal Fat Pro Carbs

B ______
L ______
S ______
D ______

DAY 16: **MON TUES WED THU FRI SAT SUN** Cal Fat Pro Carbs

B ______
L ______
S ______
D ______

DAY 17: **MON TUES WED THU FRI SAT SUN** Cal Fat Pro Carbs

B ______
L ______
S ______
D ______

DAY 18: **MON TUES WED THU FRI SAT SUN** Cal Fat Pro Carbs

B ______
L ______
S ______
D ______

DAY 19: **MON TUES WED THU FRI SAT SUN** Cal Fat Pro Carbs

B ______
L ______
S ______
D ______

DAY 20: **MON TUES WED THU FRI SAT SUN** Cal Fat Pro Carbs

B ______
L ______
S ______
D ______

DAY 21: **MON TUES WED THU FRI SAT SUN** Cal Fat Pro Carbs

B ______
L ______
S ______
D ______

DAY 15: **MON TUES WED THU FRI SAT SUN** *Time* *Calories Burned*

Exercise ______

Water ______ Steps ______

Sleep ______ Weight ______

Stress Level 0 1 2 3 4 5 6 7 8 9 10 11

DAY 16: **MON TUES WED THU FRI SAT SUN** *Time* *Calories Burned*

Exercise ______

Water ______ Steps ______

Sleep ______ Weight ______

Stress Level 0 1 2 3 4 5 6 7 8 9 10 11

DAY 17: **MON TUES WED THU FRI SAT SUN** *Time* *Calories Burned*

Exercise ______

Water ______ Steps ______

Sleep ______ Weight ______

Stress Level 0 1 2 3 4 5 6 7 8 9 10 11

DAY 18: **MON TUES WED THU FRI SAT SUN** *Time* *Calories Burned*

Exercise ______

Water ______ Steps ______

Sleep ______ Weight ______

Stress Level 0 1 2 3 4 5 6 7 8 9 10 11

DAY 19: **MON TUES WED THU FRI SAT SUN** *Time* *Calories Burned*

Exercise ______

Water ______ Steps ______

Sleep ______ Weight ______

Stress Level 0 1 2 3 4 5 6 7 8 9 10 11

DAY 20: **MON TUES WED THU FRI SAT SUN** *Time* *Calories Burned*

Exercise ______

Water ______ Steps ______

Sleep ______ Weight ______

Stress Level 0 1 2 3 4 5 6 7 8 9 10 11

DAY 21: **MON TUES WED THU FRI SAT SUN** *Time* *Calories Burned*

Exercise ______

Water ______ Steps ______

Sleep ______ Weight ______

Stress Level 0 1 2 3 4 5 6 7 8 9 10 11

MEAL PLANNER * MONTH ______ YR ____

DAY 22: MON TUES WED THU FRI SAT SUN Cal Fat Pro Carbs

B ______
L ______
S ______
D ______

DAY 23: MON TUES WED THU FRI SAT SUN Cal Fat Pro Carbs

B ______
L ______
S ______
D ______

DAY 24: MON TUES WED THU FRI SAT SUN Cal Fat Pro Carbs

B ______
L ______
S ______
D ______

DAY 25: MON TUES WED THU FRI SAT SUN Cal Fat Pro Carbs

B ______
L ______
S ______
D ______

DAY 26: MON TUES WED THU FRI SAT SUN Cal Fat Pro Carbs

B ______
L ______
S ______
D ______

DAY 27: MON TUES WED THU FRI SAT SUN Cal Fat Pro Carbs

B ______
L ______
S ______
D ______

DAY 28: MON TUES WED THU FRI SAT SUN Cal Fat Pro Carbs

B ______
L ______
S ______
D ______

DAY 22: **MON TUES WED THU FRI SAT SUN** *Time* *Calories Burned*

Exercise ______

Water ______ Steps ______

Sleep ______ Weight ______

Stress Level 0 1 2 3 4 5 6 7 8 9 10 11

DAY 23: **MON TUES WED THU FRI SAT SUN** *Time* *Calories Burned*

Exercise ______

Water ______ Steps ______

Sleep ______ Weight ______

Stress Level 0 1 2 3 4 5 6 7 8 9 10 11

DAY 24: **MON TUES WED THU FRI SAT SUN** *Time* *Calories Burned*

Exercise ______

Water ______ Steps ______

Sleep ______ Weight ______

Stress Level 0 1 2 3 4 5 6 7 8 9 10 11

DAY 25: **MON TUES WED THU FRI SAT SUN** *Time* *Calories Burned*

Exercise ______

Water ______ Steps ______

Sleep ______ Weight ______

Stress Level 0 1 2 3 4 5 6 7 8 9 10 11

DAY 26: **MON TUES WED THU FRI SAT SUN** *Time* *Calories Burned*

Exercise ______

Water ______ Steps ______

Sleep ______ Weight ______

Stress Level 0 1 2 3 4 5 6 7 8 9 10 11

DAY 27: **MON TUES WED THU FRI SAT SUN** *Time* *Calories Burned*

Exercise ______

Water ______ Steps ______

Sleep ______ Weight ______

Stress Level 0 1 2 3 4 5 6 7 8 9 10 11

DAY 28: **MON TUES WED THU FRI SAT SUN** *Time* *Calories Burned*

Exercise ______

Water ______ Steps ______

Sleep ______ Weight ______

Stress Level 0 1 2 3 4 5 6 7 8 9 10 11

DAY 29: **MON TUES WED THU FRI SAT SUN** Cal Fat Pro Carbs

B ____

L ____

S ____

D ____

DAY 30: **MON TUES WED THU FRI SAT SUN** Cal Fat Pro Carbs

B ____

L ____

S ____

D ____

DAY 31: **MON TUES WED THU FRI SAT SUN** Cal Fat Pro Carbs

B ____

L ____

S ____

D ____

GOALS

	Achieved Y	N
1. ____	☐	☐
2. ____	☐	☐
3. ____	☐	☐
4. ____	☐	☐
5. ____	☐	☐

End of Month Results

Weight

Blood Pressure

Resting Heart Rate

DAY 29: **MON TUES WED THU FRI SAT SUN** *Time* *Calories Burned*

Exercise ______________________

Water ______________ Steps ______________

Sleep ______________ Weight ______________

Stress Level 0 1 2 3 4 5 6 7 8 9 10 11

DAY 30: **MON TUES WED THU FRI SAT SUN** *Time* *Calories Burned*

Exercise ______________________

Water ______________ Steps ______________

Sleep ______________ Weight ______________

Stress Level 0 1 2 3 4 5 6 7 8 9 10 11

DAY 31: **MON TUES WED THU FRI SAT SUN** *Time* *Calories Burned*

Exercise ______________________

Water ______________ Steps ______________

Sleep ______________ Weight ______________

Stress Level 0 1 2 3 4 5 6 7 8 9 10 11

STRESSORS

Resolved Y N

1. ______________________ ☐ ☐
2. ______________________ ☐ ☐
3. ______________________ ☐ ☐
4. ______________________ ☐ ☐
5. ______________________ ☐ ☐

# of Successful Days

Count all the days this month you achieved your own health goals.

Exercise ◯ Water ◯ Steps ◯ Sleep ◯ Weight ◯

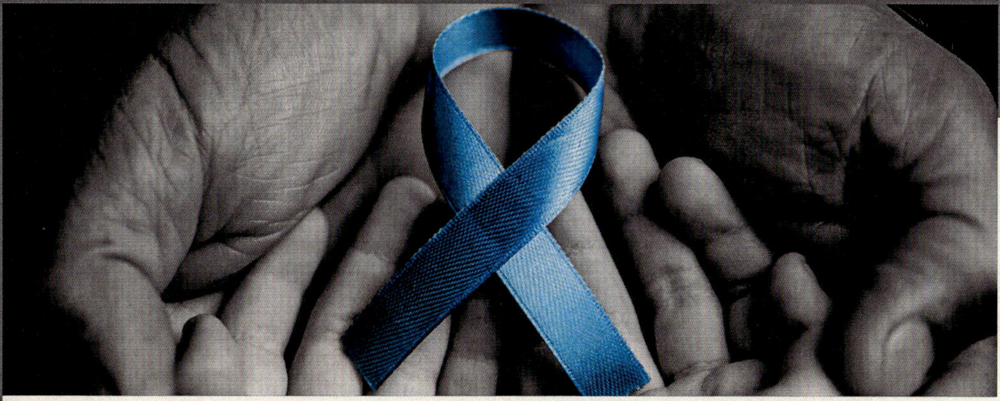

11. CANCER

Breast, Colon, Lung, Prostate, Leukemia, Skin, Lymphoma

Trauma and shock manifest in the body as cancer. Many of the foods we eat, especially meat, contain cancerous cells. Once these cells get into the human body, they replicate. Most animals are killed in an inhumane way, so that trauma gets passed on to the person consuming it. Also, if an individual experiences sudden traumatic events, doesn't express it, doesn't forgive, holds resentment, those emotions can produce cancer.

Set some goals for the month, and at the end, we will reflect on your progress. You can track your meals, exercise, appointments, and weight goals. Set some spiritual goals too.

GOALS

1. ____________________
2. ____________________
3. ____________________
4. ____________________
5. ____________________

> *"For which cause we faint not; but though our outward man perish, yet the inward man is renewed day by day. For our light affliction, which is but for a moment, worketh for us a far more exceeding and eternal weight of glory;"*
>
> *2 Corinthians 4:16, 17*

Monthly Affirmation:

"I am a compassionate, loving person."

Exercise: *Spend time in nature, on purpose. Look at every living thing, plant, human, animal. Love them.*

FOODS to Reduce **Cancer Risk:**

- **Beans:** Black, Navy, Pinto, Dried
- **Fat:** Avocado Oil, Macadamia Nut Oil, Algae Oil
- **Fruit:** Black Raspberries, Tomatoes, Grapefruit, Cherries
- **Herb:** Garlic, Elderberry, Soursop, Basil, Parsley
- **Protein:** Tofu, Plant Protein, Wild Salmon, Cold-Water Fish
- **Nuts:** Walnuts, Pine Nuts, Brazil
- **Root:** Rutabaga, Turnips, Carrot, Sweet Potato
- **Vegetables:** Broccoli, Cauliflower, Cabbage, Kale, Squash, Peppers
- **Vitamins:** A, C, E, Beta-Carotene
- **Grains:** Flaxseed, Chia, Millet, Buckwheat

JUICE to Reduce **Cancer Risk:**

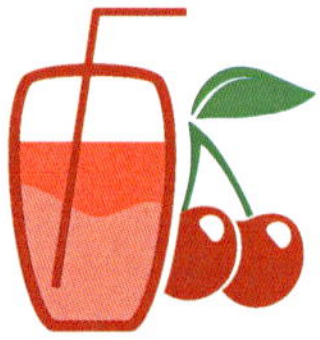

Elderberry
Soursop
Cherries

Contact Vandene:
for Local South Florida Delivery
ordersmavis@gmail.com

M.A.V.I.S
Health Drinks

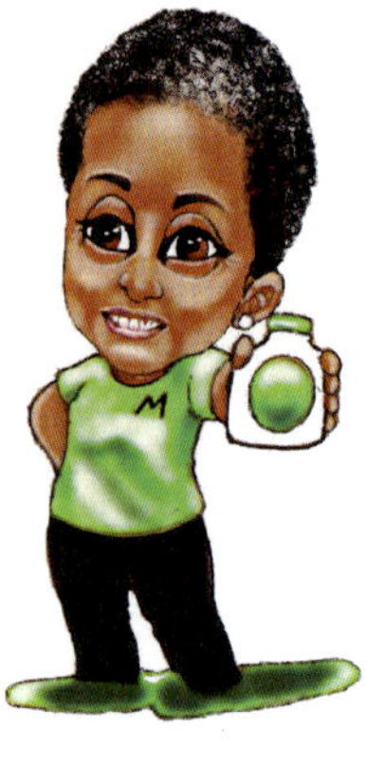

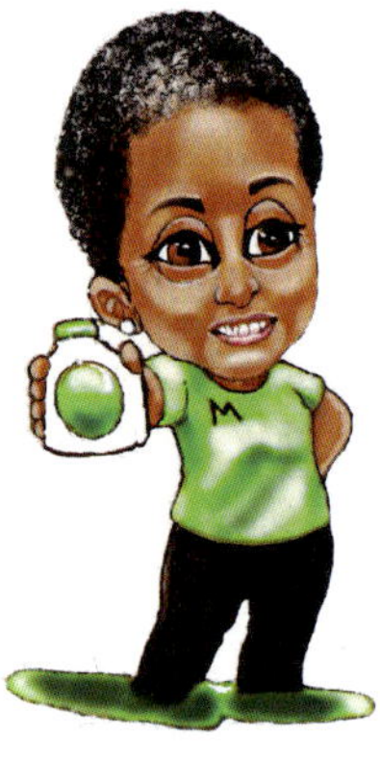

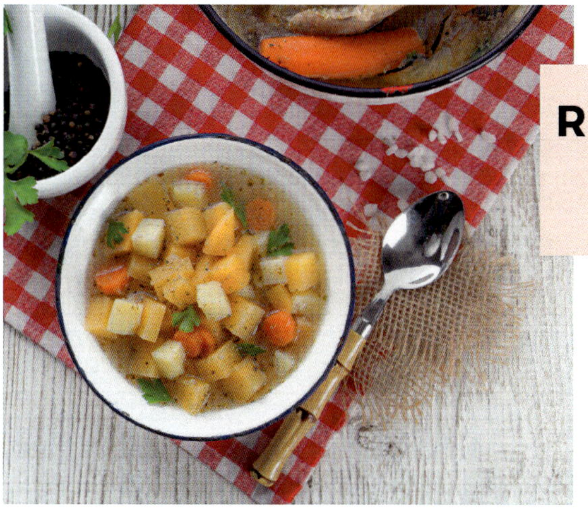

ROOT VEGETABLE
SOUP W/ CHICKEN

YIELDS 2 SERVINGS

TOTAL TIME: 35 MINS

1- tbsp Avocado Oil
2 - cloves of Garlic cloves
2 - cups of Vegetable Broth
1/2 - can of Black Beans, rinsed
1/4 - cup Lentils
1 - Celery, sliced thin
1/4 - cups Carrots, diced
1/4 - cup of Rutabaga, cubed
1/4 - cup of Onion, chopped
1/4 - cup of Squash, chopped
1/4 - cup Sweet Potato, cubed
1/4 - cup of Cauliflower, chopped
1 - tsp of Oregano, chopped
1 - tsp of Basil, chopped
2 - Bay leaves

DIRECTIONS:

- Heat a large pot to Medium-high
- Add oil to pot
- Add Onions, Carrots, Celery, Rutabaga, Squash
- Cook for 5 minutes, then add Garlic
- Stir in Vegetable Broth
- Add Lentils, Black Beans, Bay Leaves
- Bring to a boil, then reduce to simmer
- Cook for 10 minutes
- Add Sweet Potato, Cauliflower
- Cook for 10 minutes
- Stir in Oregano and Basil
- Cook for 5 more minutes, remove bay leaves
- Serve with torn parsley leaves (optional)

Medical Appointments

Date/Time Office

____

____

____

____

MEAL PLANNER * MONTH ______ YR ____

DAY 1: **MON TUES WED THU FRI SAT SUN** Cal Fat Pro Carbs

B ____

L ____

S ____

D ____

DAY 2: **MON TUES WED THU FRI SAT SUN** Cal Fat Pro Carbs

B ____

L ____

S ____

D ____

DAY 3: **MON TUES WED THU FRI SAT SUN** Cal Fat Pro Carbs

B ____

L ____

S ____

D ____

DAY 4: **MON TUES WED THU FRI SAT SUN** Cal Fat Pro Carbs

B ____

L ____

S ____

D ____

DAY 5: **MON TUES WED THU FRI SAT SUN** Cal Fat Pro Carbs

B ____

L ____

S ____

D ____

DAY 6: **MON TUES WED THU FRI SAT SUN** Cal Fat Pro Carbs

B ____

L ____

S ____

D ____

DAY 7: **MON TUES WED THU FRI SAT SUN** Cal Fat Pro Carbs

B ____

L ____

S ____

D ____

ACTIVITY PLANNER * MONTH ________ YR ____

DAY 1: **MON TUES WED THU FRI SAT SUN** *Time* *Calories Burned*

Exercise ______________________________

Water ______________ Steps ______________

Sleep ______________ Weight ______________

Stress Level 0 1 2 3 4 5 6 7 8 9 10 11

DAY 2: **MON TUES WED THU FRI SAT SUN** *Time* *Calories Burned*

Exercise ______________________________

Water ______________ Steps ______________

Sleep ______________ Weight ______________

Stress Level 0 1 2 3 4 5 6 7 8 9 10 11

DAY 3: **MON TUES WED THU FRI SAT SUN** *Time* *Calories Burned*

Exercise ______________________________

Water ______________ Steps ______________

Sleep ______________ Weight ______________

Stress Level 0 1 2 3 4 5 6 7 8 9 10 11

DAY 4: **MON TUES WED THU FRI SAT SUN** *Time* *Calories Burned*

Exercise ______________________________

Water ______________ Steps ______________

Sleep ______________ Weight ______________

Stress Level 0 1 2 3 4 5 6 7 8 9 10 11

DAY 5: **MON TUES WED THU FRI SAT SUN** *Time* *Calories Burned*

Exercise ______________________________

Water ______________ Steps ______________

Sleep ______________ Weight ______________

Stress Level 0 1 2 3 4 5 6 7 8 9 10 11

DAY 6: **MON TUES WED THU FRI SAT SUN** *Time* *Calories Burned*

Exercise ______________________________

Water ______________ Steps ______________

Sleep ______________ Weight ______________

Stress Level 0 1 2 3 4 5 6 7 8 9 10 11

DAY 7: **MON TUES WED THU FRI SAT SUN** *Time* *Calories Burned*

Exercise ______________________________

Water ______________ Steps ______________

Sleep ______________ Weight ______________

Stress Level 0 1 2 3 4 5 6 7 8 9 10 11

DAY 8: **MON TUES WED THU FRI SAT SUN** Cal Fat Pro Carbs

B ____________________

L ____________________

S ____________________

D ____________________

DAY 9: **MON TUES WED THU FRI SAT SUN** Cal Fat Pro Carbs

B ____________________

L ____________________

S ____________________

D ____________________

DAY 10: **MON TUES WED THU FRI SAT SUN** Cal Fat Pro Carbs

B ____________________

L ____________________

S ____________________

D ____________________

DAY 11: **MON TUES WED THU FRI SAT SUN** Cal Fat Pro Carbs

B ____________________

L ____________________

S ____________________

D ____________________

DAY 12: **MON TUES WED THU FRI SAT SUN** Cal Fat Pro Carbs

B ____________________

L ____________________

S ____________________

D ____________________

DAY 13: **MON TUES WED THU FRI SAT SUN** Cal Fat Pro Carbs

B ____________________

L ____________________

S ____________________

D ____________________

DAY 14: **MON TUES WED THU FRI SAT SUN** Cal Fat Pro Carbs

B ____________________

L ____________________

S ____________________

D ____________________

DAY 8: **MON TUES WED THU FRI SAT SUN** *Time* *Calories Burned*

Exercise ______________________________

Water ____________ Steps ____________

Sleep ____________ Weight ____________

Stress Level 0 1 2 3 4 5 6 7 8 9 10 11

DAY 9: **MON TUES WED THU FRI SAT SUN** *Time* *Calories Burned*

Exercise ______________________________

Water ____________ Steps ____________

Sleep ____________ Weight ____________

Stress Level 0 1 2 3 4 5 6 7 8 9 10 11

DAY 10: **MON TUES WED THU FRI SAT SUN** *Time* *Calories Burned*

Exercise ______________________________

Water ____________ Steps ____________

Sleep ____________ Weight ____________

Stress Level 0 1 2 3 4 5 6 7 8 9 10 11

DAY 11: **MON TUES WED THU FRI SAT SUN** *Time* *Calories Burned*

Exercise ______________________________

Water ____________ Steps ____________

Sleep ____________ Weight ____________

Stress Level 0 1 2 3 4 5 6 7 8 9 10 11

DAY 12: **MON TUES WED THU FRI SAT SUN** *Time* *Calories Burned*

Exercise ______________________________

Water ____________ Steps ____________

Sleep ____________ Weight ____________

Stress Level 0 1 2 3 4 5 6 7 8 9 10 11

DAY 13: **MON TUES WED THU FRI SAT SUN** *Time* *Calories Burned*

Exercise ______________________________

Water ____________ Steps ____________

Sleep ____________ Weight ____________

Stress Level 0 1 2 3 4 5 6 7 8 9 10 11

DAY 14: **MON TUES WED THU FRI SAT SUN** *Time* *Calories Burned*

Exercise ______________________________

Water ____________ Steps ____________

Sleep ____________ Weight ____________

Stress Level 0 1 2 3 4 5 6 7 8 9 10 11

MEAL PLANNER * MONTH ______ YR ____

DAY 15: **MON TUES WED THU FRI SAT SUN** Cal Fat Pro Carbs

B

L

S

D

DAY 16: **MON TUES WED THU FRI SAT SUN** Cal Fat Pro Carbs

B

L

S

D

DAY 17: **MON TUES WED THU FRI SAT SUN** Cal Fat Pro Carbs

B

L

S

D

DAY 18: **MON TUES WED THU FRI SAT SUN** Cal Fat Pro Carbs

B

L

S

D

DAY 19: **MON TUES WED THU FRI SAT SUN** Cal Fat Pro Carbs

B

L

S

D

DAY 20: **MON TUES WED THU FRI SAT SUN** Cal Fat Pro Carbs

B

L

S

D

DAY 21: **MON TUES WED THU FRI SAT SUN** Cal Fat Pro Carbs

B

L

S

D

DAY 15: **MON TUES WED THU FRI SAT SUN** *Time* *Calories Burned*

Exercise ______

Water ______ Steps ______

Sleep ______ Weight ______

Stress Level 0 1 2 3 4 5 6 7 8 9 10 11

DAY 16: **MON TUES WED THU FRI SAT SUN** *Time* *Calories Burned*

Exercise ______

Water ______ Steps ______

Sleep ______ Weight ______

Stress Level 0 1 2 3 4 5 6 7 8 9 10 11

DAY 17: **MON TUES WED THU FRI SAT SUN** *Time* *Calories Burned*

Exercise ______

Water ______ Steps ______

Sleep ______ Weight ______

Stress Level 0 1 2 3 4 5 6 7 8 9 10 11

DAY 18: **MON TUES WED THU FRI SAT SUN** *Time* *Calories Burned*

Exercise ______

Water ______ Steps ______

Sleep ______ Weight ______

Stress Level 0 1 2 3 4 5 6 7 8 9 10 11

DAY 19: **MON TUES WED THU FRI SAT SUN** *Time* *Calories Burned*

Exercise ______

Water ______ Steps ______

Sleep ______ Weight ______

Stress Level 0 1 2 3 4 5 6 7 8 9 10 11

DAY 20: **MON TUES WED THU FRI SAT SUN** *Time* *Calories Burned*

Exercise ______

Water ______ Steps ______

Sleep ______ Weight ______

Stress Level 0 1 2 3 4 5 6 7 8 9 10 11

DAY 21: **MON TUES WED THU FRI SAT SUN** *Time* *Calories Burned*

Exercise ______

Water ______ Steps ______

Sleep ______ Weight ______

Stress Level 0 1 2 3 4 5 6 7 8 9 10 11

MEAL PLANNER * MONTH ________ YR ____

DAY 22: MON TUES WED THU FRI SAT SUN Cal Fat Pro Carbs

B ____
L ____
S ____
D ____

DAY 23: MON TUES WED THU FRI SAT SUN Cal Fat Pro Carbs

B ____
L ____
S ____
D ____

DAY 24: MON TUES WED THU FRI SAT SUN Cal Fat Pro Carbs

B ____
L ____
S ____
D ____

DAY 25: MON TUES WED THU FRI SAT SUN Cal Fat Pro Carbs

B ____
L ____
S ____
D ____

DAY 26: MON TUES WED THU FRI SAT SUN Cal Fat Pro Carbs

B ____
L ____
S ____
D ____

DAY 27: MON TUES WED THU FRI SAT SUN Cal Fat Pro Carbs

B ____
L ____
S ____
D ____

DAY 28: MON TUES WED THU FRI SAT SUN Cal Fat Pro Carbs

B ____
L ____
S ____
D ____

DAY 22: **MON TUES WED THU FRI SAT SUN** *Time* *Calories Burned*

Exercise ____________________

Water ____________ Steps ____________

Sleep ____________ Weight ____________

Stress Level 0 1 2 3 4 5 6 7 8 9 10 11

DAY 23: **MON TUES WED THU FRI SAT SUN** *Time* *Calories Burned*

Exercise ____________________

Water ____________ Steps ____________

Sleep ____________ Weight ____________

Stress Level 0 1 2 3 4 5 6 7 8 9 10 11

DAY 24: **MON TUES WED THU FRI SAT SUN** *Time* *Calories Burned*

Exercise ____________________

Water ____________ Steps ____________

Sleep ____________ Weight ____________

Stress Level 0 1 2 3 4 5 6 7 8 9 10 11

DAY 25: **MON TUES WED THU FRI SAT SUN** *Time* *Calories Burned*

Exercise ____________________

Water ____________ Steps ____________

Sleep ____________ Weight ____________

Stress Level 0 1 2 3 4 5 6 7 8 9 10 11

DAY 26: **MON TUES WED THU FRI SAT SUN** *Time* *Calories Burned*

Exercise ____________________

Water ____________ Steps ____________

Sleep ____________ Weight ____________

Stress Level 0 1 2 3 4 5 6 7 8 9 10 11

DAY 27: **MON TUES WED THU FRI SAT SUN** *Time* *Calories Burned*

Exercise ____________________

Water ____________ Steps ____________

Sleep ____________ Weight ____________

Stress Level 0 1 2 3 4 5 6 7 8 9 10 11

DAY 28: **MON TUES WED THU FRI SAT SUN** *Time* *Calories Burned*

Exercise ____________________

Water ____________ Steps ____________

Sleep ____________ Weight ____________

Stress Level 0 1 2 3 4 5 6 7 8 9 10 11

MEAL PLANNER * MONTH ________ YR ____

DAY 29: **MON TUES WED THU FRI SAT SUN** Cal Fat Pro Carbs

B ____
L ____
S ____
D ____

DAY 30: **MON TUES WED THU FRI SAT SUN** Cal Fat Pro Carbs

B ____
L ____
S ____
D ____

DAY 31: **MON TUES WED THU FRI SAT SUN** Cal Fat Pro Carbs

B ____
L ____
S ____
D ____

GOALS

	Achieved Y	N
1. ____	☐	☐
2. ____	☐	☐
3. ____	☐	☐
4. ____	☐	☐
5. ____	☐	☐

End of Month Results

Weight

Blood Pressure

Resting Heart Rate

DAY 29: **MON TUES WED THU FRI SAT SUN** *Time* *Calories Burned*

Exercise ______________________________

Water ______________ Steps ______________

Sleep ______________ Weight ______________

Stress Level 0 1 2 3 4 5 6 7 8 9 10 11

DAY 30: **MON TUES WED THU FRI SAT SUN** *Time* *Calories Burned*

Exercise ______________________________

Water ______________ Steps ______________

Sleep ______________ Weight ______________

Stress Level 0 1 2 3 4 5 6 7 8 9 10 11

DAY 31: **MON TUES WED THU FRI SAT SUN** *Time* *Calories Burned*

Exercise ______________________________

Water ______________ Steps ______________

Sleep ______________ Weight ______________

Stress Level 0 1 2 3 4 5 6 7 8 9 10 11

STRESSORS

	Resolved Y	Resolved N
1. ______________	☐	☐
2. ______________	☐	☐
3. ______________	☐	☐
4. ______________	☐	☐
5. ______________	☐	☐

of Successful Days

Count all the days this month you achieved your own health goals.

Exercise Water Steps Sleep Weight

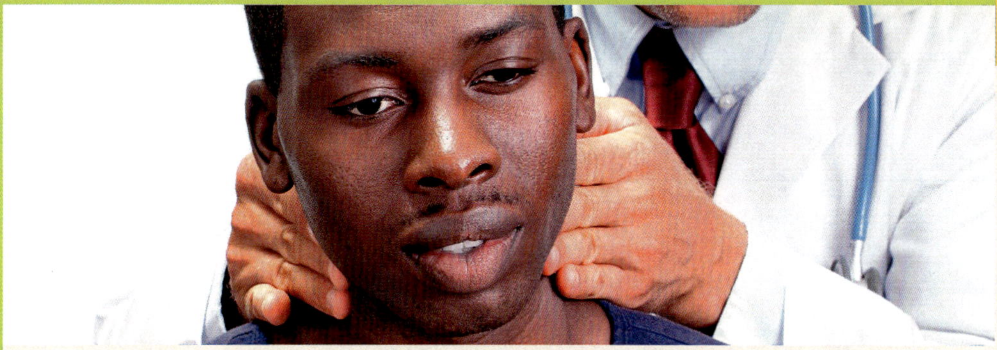

12. LYMPH

Immune System: White Blood Cells, Bone Marrow, Thymus Lymph Nodes, Spleen, Tonsils, Mucous Membrane

Most doctors only get 30 minutes of training on the Lymphatic system in medical school . The lymphatic system cleans the blood. Toxins go there to die. When the lymph nodes get blocked, toxins bunch up, create infections and mutate. The spiritual cause of lymph blockage and malfunction is the feeling of not being protected, threatened, and unable to defend one's self. Each node represents a different cause. Nodes are found in the neck, armpits, legs, groin, stomach, breast. Research your lymphatic system, because your doctor has not. Movement makes the lymphatic system flow, it does not move on its own. The blood moves by the pumping of the heart. The lymph becomes a stagnant pool when sedentary. Deodorants contain aluminum, which block the lymph nodes and cause cancer around the breasts and armpits. Detergent is toxic. Do your research!

Set some goals for the month, and at the end, we will reflect on your progress. You can track your meals, exercise, appointments, and weight goals. Set some spiritual goals too.

GOALS

1. ______________________________
2. ______________________________
3. ______________________________
4. ______________________________
5. ______________________________

> *"Having purified your souls by your obedience to the truth for a sincere brotherly love, love one another earnestly from a pure heart, since you have been born again, not of perishable seed but of imperishable, through the living and abiding word of God;"*
>
> *1 Peter 1:22*

Monthly Affirmation:

"I am constantly moving forward on my path."

Exercise: *Give yourself a massage, either your feet, your hands, your neck, your legs. Move your lymph.*

FOODS to Improve Lymph Flow:

- **Beans:** Fava, Lima, Northern, Peas
- **Oil:** Poke Root Oil, Chlorophyll
- **Fruit:** Cranberries, Avocado, Kiwi, Banana, Papaya, Lemon, Lime
- **Herb:** Arctic Root, Rose Root, Red Clover, Siberian Ginseng, Turmeric
- **Protein:** Dark meat Chicken, Turkey
- **Nuts:** Walnuts, Almonds, Brazil Nuts, Pumpkin Seed
- **Root:** Garlic, Beets, Potatoes
- **Vegetables:** Dandelion, Green and Red Peppers, Broccoli, Spinach, Seaweed
- **Vitamins:** A, C, K, Iron, Zinc, Magnesium
- **Grains:** Flaxseed, Chia, Hemp, Iodine, Buckwheat

JUICE to Improve Lymph Flow:

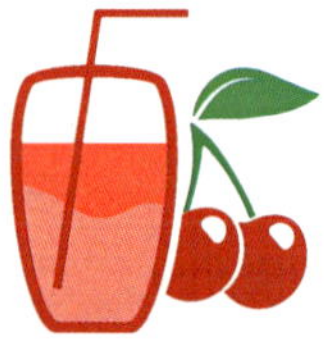

Cranberry
Spinach
Orange

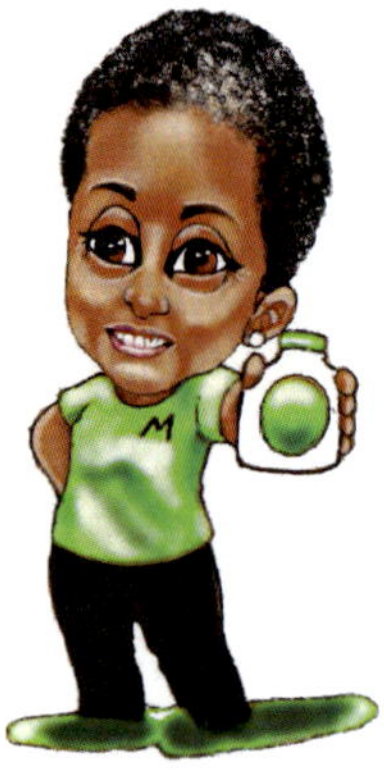

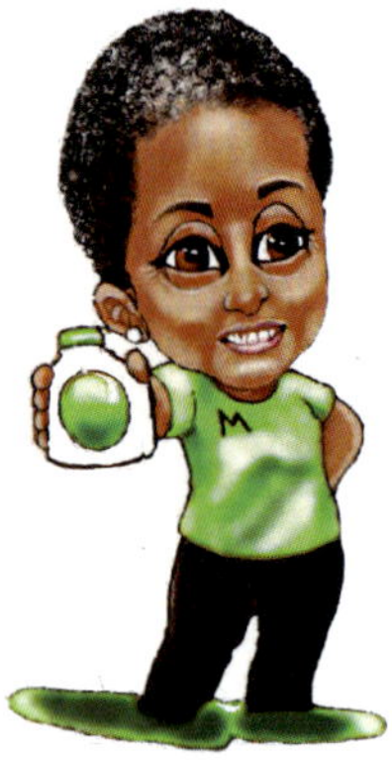

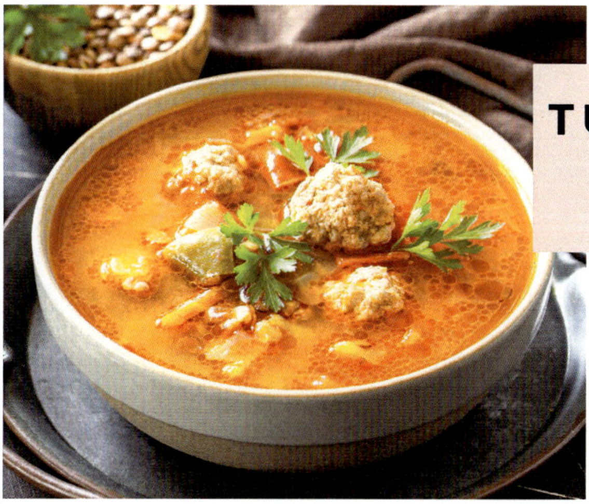

TURKEY MEATBALL
SOUP W/ BROCCOLI

YIELDS 2 -3 SERVINGS

TOTAL TIME: 30 MINS

1 - 12 oz. Bag of Turkey Meatballs (Fully-cooked)
1 - Ginger piece, peeled and grated
2 - Carrots, peeled and chopped
1 - Zucchini, chopped
1 - Bunch of Broccolini , chopped
3 - cups of Vegetable Broth
1 - cup of Coconut Milk
1 - Yellow Onion, chopped
3 - Cloves of Garlic, minced
1 - tbsp of Avocado oil (or other oil)
1 - tsp of Ground Turmeric
2 - tsp of Worcestershire sauce
2 - tsp of Lime juice
1 - tsp of Sea salt

DIRECTIONS:

- Heat the oil in a large pot over Medium-heat
- Add the Onion and Garlic, stirring occasionally
- Grill for 3 minutes.
- Add the turkey meatballs. Grill both sides
- Add all remaining ingredients, stir and cover
- Bring soup to a boil, then reduce to a simmer
- Cook for 15 - 20 minutes
- Taste the soup for flavor, and season to taste
- Serve with croutons or Almond-flour crackers

Medical Appointments

Date/Time	Office

MEAL PLANNER * MONTH ________ YR ______

DAY 1: MON TUES WED THU FRI SAT SUN Cal Fat Pro Carbs

B ______

L ______

S ______

D ______

DAY 2: MON TUES WED THU FRI SAT SUN Cal Fat Pro Carbs

B ______

L ______

S ______

D ______

DAY 3: MON TUES WED THU FRI SAT SUN Cal Fat Pro Carbs

B ______

L ______

S ______

D ______

DAY 4: MON TUES WED THU FRI SAT SUN Cal Fat Pro Carbs

B ______

L ______

S ______

D ______

DAY 5: MON TUES WED THU FRI SAT SUN Cal Fat Pro Carbs

B ______

L ______

S ______

D ______

DAY 6: MON TUES WED THU FRI SAT SUN Cal Fat Pro Carbs

B ______

L ______

S ______

D ______

DAY 7: MON TUES WED THU FRI SAT SUN Cal Fat Pro Carbs

B ______

L ______

S ______

D ______

ACTIVITY PLANNER * MONTH __________ YR ____

DAY 1: **MON TUES WED THU FRI SAT SUN** *Time* *Calories Burned*

Exercise ____

Water ____________________ Steps ____________________

Sleep ____________________ Weight ____________________

Stress Level 0 1 2 3 4 5 6 7 8 9 10 11

DAY 2: **MON TUES WED THU FRI SAT SUN** *Time* *Calories Burned*

Exercise ____

Water ____________________ Steps ____________________

Sleep ____________________ Weight ____________________

Stress Level 0 1 2 3 4 5 6 7 8 9 10 11

DAY 3: **MON TUES WED THU FRI SAT SUN** *Time* *Calories Burned*

Exercise ____

Water ____________________ Steps ____________________

Sleep ____________________ Weight ____________________

Stress Level 0 1 2 3 4 5 6 7 8 9 10 11

DAY 4: **MON TUES WED THU FRI SAT SUN** *Time* *Calories Burned*

Exercise ____

Water ____________________ Steps ____________________

Sleep ____________________ Weight ____________________

Stress Level 0 1 2 3 4 5 6 7 8 9 10 11

DAY 5: **MON TUES WED THU FRI SAT SUN** *Time* *Calories Burned*

Exercise ____

Water ____________________ Steps ____________________

Sleep ____________________ Weight ____________________

Stress Level 0 1 2 3 4 5 6 7 8 9 10 11

DAY 6: **MON TUES WED THU FRI SAT SUN** *Time* *Calories Burned*

Exercise ____

Water ____________________ Steps ____________________

Sleep ____________________ Weight ____________________

Stress Level 0 1 2 3 4 5 6 7 8 9 10 11

DAY 7: **MON TUES WED THU FRI SAT SUN** *Time* *Calories Burned*

Exercise ____

Water ____________________ Steps ____________________

Sleep ____________________ Weight ____________________

Stress Level 0 1 2 3 4 5 6 7 8 9 10 11

MEAL PLANNER * MONTH ______ YR ______

DAY 8: **MON TUES WED THU FRI SAT SUN** Cal Fat Pro Carbs

B ____________________

L ____________________

S ____________________

D ____________________

DAY 9: **MON TUES WED THU FRI SAT SUN** Cal Fat Pro Carbs

B ____________________

L ____________________

S ____________________

D ____________________

DAY 10: **MON TUES WED THU FRI SAT SUN** Cal Fat Pro Carbs

B ____________________

L ____________________

S ____________________

D ____________________

DAY 11: **MON TUES WED THU FRI SAT SUN** Cal Fat Pro Carbs

B ____________________

L ____________________

S ____________________

D ____________________

DAY 12: **MON TUES WED THU FRI SAT SUN** Cal Fat Pro Carbs

B ____________________

L ____________________

S ____________________

D ____________________

DAY 13: **MON TUES WED THU FRI SAT SUN** Cal Fat Pro Carbs

B ____________________

L ____________________

S ____________________

D ____________________

DAY 14: **MON TUES WED THU FRI SAT SUN** Cal Fat Pro Carbs

B ____________________

L ____________________

S ____________________

D ____________________

DAY 8: **MON TUES WED THU FRI SAT SUN** *Time* *Calories Burned*

Exercise ____________________

Water ____________ Steps ____________

Sleep ____________ Weight ____________

Stress Level 0 1 2 3 4 5 6 7 8 9 10 11

DAY 9: **MON TUES WED THU FRI SAT SUN** *Time* *Calories Burned*

Exercise ____________________

Water ____________ Steps ____________

Sleep ____________ Weight ____________

Stress Level 0 1 2 3 4 5 6 7 8 9 10 11

DAY 10: **MON TUES WED THU FRI SAT SUN** *Time* *Calories Burned*

Exercise ____________________

Water ____________ Steps ____________

Sleep ____________ Weight ____________

Stress Level 0 1 2 3 4 5 6 7 8 9 10 11

DAY 11: **MON TUES WED THU FRI SAT SUN** *Time* *Calories Burned*

Exercise ____________________

Water ____________ Steps ____________

Sleep ____________ Weight ____________

Stress Level 0 1 2 3 4 5 6 7 8 9 10 11

DAY 12: **MON TUES WED THU FRI SAT SUN** *Time* *Calories Burned*

Exercise ____________________

Water ____________ Steps ____________

Sleep ____________ Weight ____________

Stress Level 0 1 2 3 4 5 6 7 8 9 10 11

DAY 13: **MON TUES WED THU FRI SAT SUN** *Time* *Calories Burned*

Exercise ____________________

Water ____________ Steps ____________

Sleep ____________ Weight ____________

Stress Level 0 1 2 3 4 5 6 7 8 9 10 11

DAY 14: **MON TUES WED THU FRI SAT SUN** *Time* *Calories Burned*

Exercise ____________________

Water ____________ Steps ____________

Sleep ____________ Weight ____________

Stress Level 0 1 2 3 4 5 6 7 8 9 10 11

MEAL PLANNER * MONTH ________ YR ______

DAY 15: **MON TUES WED THU FRI SAT SUN** Cal Fat Pro Carbs

B ____

L ____

S ____

D ____

DAY 16: **MON TUES WED THU FRI SAT SUN** Cal Fat Pro Carbs

B ____

L ____

S ____

D ____

DAY 17: **MON TUES WED THU FRI SAT SUN** Cal Fat Pro Carbs

B ____

L ____

S ____

D ____

DAY 18: **MON TUES WED THU FRI SAT SUN** Cal Fat Pro Carbs

B ____

L ____

S ____

D ____

DAY 19: **MON TUES WED THU FRI SAT SUN** Cal Fat Pro Carbs

B ____

L ____

S ____

D ____

DAY 20: **MON TUES WED THU FRI SAT SUN** Cal Fat Pro Carbs

B ____

L ____

S ____

D ____

DAY 21: **MON TUES WED THU FRI SAT SUN** Cal Fat Pro Carbs

B ____

L ____

S ____

D ____

DAY 15: **MON TUES WED THU FRI SAT SUN** *Time* *Calories Burned*

Exercise ______

Water ______ Steps ______

Sleep ______ Weight ______

Stress Level 0 1 2 3 4 5 6 7 8 9 10 11

DAY 16: **MON TUES WED THU FRI SAT SUN** *Time* *Calories Burned*

Exercise ______

Water ______ Steps ______

Sleep ______ Weight ______

Stress Level 0 1 2 3 4 5 6 7 8 9 10 11

DAY 17: **MON TUES WED THU FRI SAT SUN** *Time* *Calories Burned*

Exercise ______

Water ______ Steps ______

Sleep ______ Weight ______

Stress Level 0 1 2 3 4 5 6 7 8 9 10 11

DAY 18: **MON TUES WED THU FRI SAT SUN** *Time* *Calories Burned*

Exercise ______

Water ______ Steps ______

Sleep ______ Weight ______

Stress Level 0 1 2 3 4 5 6 7 8 9 10 11

DAY 19: **MON TUES WED THU FRI SAT SUN** *Time* *Calories Burned*

Exercise ______

Water ______ Steps ______

Sleep ______ Weight ______

Stress Level 0 1 2 3 4 5 6 7 8 9 10 11

DAY 20: **MON TUES WED THU FRI SAT SUN** *Time* *Calories Burned*

Exercise ______

Water ______ Steps ______

Sleep ______ Weight ______

Stress Level 0 1 2 3 4 5 6 7 8 9 10 11

DAY 21: **MON TUES WED THU FRI SAT SUN** *Time* *Calories Burned*

Exercise ______

Water ______ Steps ______

Sleep ______ Weight ______

Stress Level 0 1 2 3 4 5 6 7 8 9 10 11

MEAL PLANNER * MONTH ________ YR ______

DAY 22: **MON TUES WED THU FRI SAT SUN** Cal Fat Pro Carbs

B ______

L ______

S ______

D ______

DAY 23: **MON TUES WED THU FRI SAT SUN** Cal Fat Pro Carbs

B ______

L ______

S ______

D ______

DAY 24: **MON TUES WED THU FRI SAT SUN** Cal Fat Pro Carbs

B ______

L ______

S ______

D ______

DAY 25: **MON TUES WED THU FRI SAT SUN** Cal Fat Pro Carbs

B ______

L ______

S ______

D ______

DAY 26: **MON TUES WED THU FRI SAT SUN** Cal Fat Pro Carbs

B ______

L ______

S ______

D ______

DAY 27: **MON TUES WED THU FRI SAT SUN** Cal Fat Pro Carbs

B ______

L ______

S ______

D ______

DAY 28: **MON TUES WED THU FRI SAT SUN** Cal Fat Pro Carbs

B ______

L ______

S ______

D ______

DAY 22: **MON TUES WED THU FRI SAT SUN** *Time* *Calories Burned*

Exercise ______________________

Water ______________ Steps ______________

Sleep ______________ Weight ______________

Stress Level 0 1 2 3 4 5 6 7 8 9 10 11

DAY 23: **MON TUES WED THU FRI SAT SUN** *Time* *Calories Burned*

Exercise ______________________

Water ______________ Steps ______________

Sleep ______________ Weight ______________

Stress Level 0 1 2 3 4 5 6 7 8 9 10 11

DAY 24: **MON TUES WED THU FRI SAT SUN** *Time* *Calories Burned*

Exercise ______________________

Water ______________ Steps ______________

Sleep ______________ Weight ______________

Stress Level 0 1 2 3 4 5 6 7 8 9 10 11

DAY 25: **MON TUES WED THU FRI SAT SUN** *Time* *Calories Burned*

Exercise ______________________

Water ______________ Steps ______________

Sleep ______________ Weight ______________

Stress Level 0 1 2 3 4 5 6 7 8 9 10 11

DAY 26: **MON TUES WED THU FRI SAT SUN** *Time* *Calories Burned*

Exercise ______________________

Water ______________ Steps ______________

Sleep ______________ Weight ______________

Stress Level 0 1 2 3 4 5 6 7 8 9 10 11

DAY 27: **MON TUES WED THU FRI SAT SUN** *Time* *Calories Burned*

Exercise ______________________

Water ______________ Steps ______________

Sleep ______________ Weight ______________

Stress Level 0 1 2 3 4 5 6 7 8 9 10 11

DAY 28: **MON TUES WED THU FRI SAT SUN** *Time* *Calories Burned*

Exercise ______________________

Water ______________ Steps ______________

Sleep ______________ Weight ______________

Stress Level 0 1 2 3 4 5 6 7 8 9 10 11

MEAL PLANNER * MONTH ________ YR ____

DAY 29: MON TUES WED THU FRI SAT SUN Cal Fat Pro Carbs

B ______
L ______
S ______
D ______

DAY 30: MON TUES WED THU FRI SAT SUN Cal Fat Pro Carbs

B ______
L ______
S ______
D ______

DAY 31: MON TUES WED THU FRI SAT SUN Cal Fat Pro Carbs

B ______
L ______
S ______
D ______

GOALS

Achieved Y N

1. ______ ☐ ☐
2. ______ ☐ ☐
3. ______ ☐ ☐
4. ______ ☐ ☐
5. ______ ☐ ☐

End of Month Results

Weight

Blood Pressure

Resting Heart Rate

DAY 29: **MON TUES WED THU FRI SAT SUN** *Time* *Calories Burned*

Exercise ______________________________

Water ______________ Steps ______________

Sleep ______________ Weight ______________

Stress Level 0 1 2 3 4 5 6 7 8 9 10 11

DAY 30: **MON TUES WED THU FRI SAT SUN** *Time* *Calories Burned*

Exercise ______________________________

Water ______________ Steps ______________

Sleep ______________ Weight ______________

Stress Level 0 1 2 3 4 5 6 7 8 9 10 11

DAY 31: **MON TUES WED THU FRI SAT SUN** *Time* *Calories Burned*

Exercise ______________________________

Water ______________ Steps ______________

Sleep ______________ Weight ______________

Stress Level 0 1 2 3 4 5 6 7 8 9 10 11

STRESSORS

Resolved

	Y	N
1. ______________	☐	☐
2. ______________	☐	☐
3. ______________	☐	☐
4. ______________	☐	☐
5. ______________	☐	☐

of Successful Days

Count all the days this month you achieved your own health goals.

Exercise Water Steps Sleep Weight

ACTIVITY PLANNER * MONTH ________ YR ____

YOU DID IT!

Let me know how well you did!! Join the conversation!

JOIN THE FACEBOOK COMMUNITY

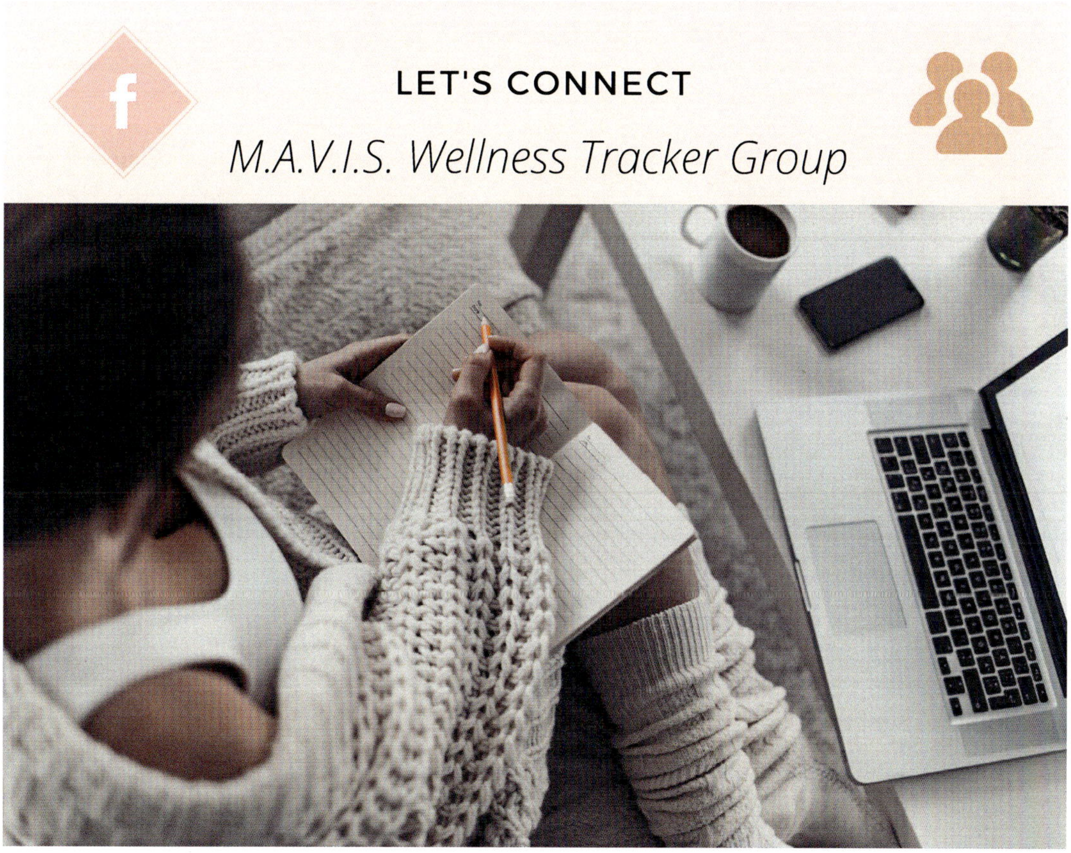

Made in United States
North Haven, CT
05 December 2023

45133168R10097